Cardiovascular System

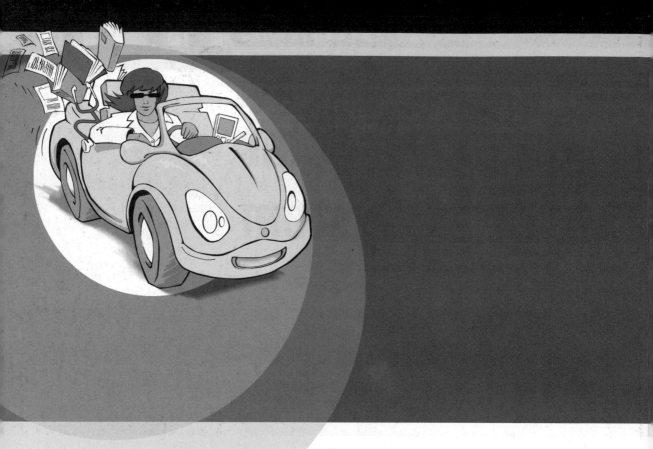

First and second edition authors:

Romeshan Suntheswaran

Toby Fagan

CRASH COURSE

Third Edition

Cardiovascular System

Series editor
Daniel Horton-Szar
BSc (Hons), MBBS (Hons), MRCGP
Northgate Medical Practice
Canterbury
Kent, UK

Faculty advisor
Professor David Newby
BA, BSc(Hons), PhD BM, DM FRCP
Professor of Cardiology and
Consultant Cardiologist,
Centre for Cardiovascular Sciences,
University of Edinburgh, Royal Infirmary,
Edinburgh, UK

Paul Sutton BMedSci (Hons)
Medical Student
University of Nottingham
UK

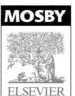

Edinburgh • London • New York • Oxford • Philadelphia • St Louis • Sydney • Toronto 2008

Commissioning Editor:	**Alison Taylor**
Development Editor:	**Kim Benson**
Project Manager:	**Frances Affleck**
Senior Designer:	**Sarah Russell**
Cover:	**Stewart Larking**
Icon illustrations:	**Geo Parkin**
Illustration Management:	**Bruce Hogarth**

© 1998, Mosby International Ltd
© 2002, Elsevier Science Ltd
© 2008, Elsevier Limited. All rights reserved.

First edition 1998
Second edition 2002
Third edition 2008

ISBN-13: 978-0-7234-3430-6

British Library Cataloguing in Publication Data
A catalogue record for this book is available from the British Library

Library of Congress Cataloging in Publication Data
A catalog record for this book is available from the Library of Congress

Note
Knowledge and best practice in this field are constantly changing. As new research and experience broaden our knowledge, changes in practice, treatment and drug therapy may become necessary or appropriate. Readers are advised to check the most current information provided (i) on procedures featured or (ii) by the manufacturer of each product to be administered, to verify the recommended dose or formula, the method and duration of administration, and contraindications. It is the responsibility of the practitioner, relying on their own experience and knowledge of the patient, to make diagnoses, to determine dosages and the best treatment for each individual patient, and to take all appropriate safety precautions. To the fullest extent of the law, neither the Publisher nor the Author assumes any liability for any injury and/or damage to persons or property arising out of or related to any use of the material contained in this book.
The Publisher

Working together to grow
libraries in developing countries

www.elsevier.com | www.bookaid.org | www.sabre.org

ELSEVIER   BOOK AID International   Sabre Foundation

The
publisher's
policy is to use
**paper manufactured
from sustainable forests**

Printed in China

Preface

My friends and colleagues will know that I'm a huge believer in the Crash Course series, and it's been a pleasure writing this book. I believe that a sound understanding of the basics, of both the sciences underpinning medicine and indeed clinical medicine itself, is the way in which to succeed at medical school.

Cardiovascular anatomy and physiology are often dreaded by preclinical medical students, usually because many text books used by undergraduates succeed in complicating even the simplest of concepts. Nonetheless, it is fundamental in your development as a doctor, as a knowledge of the pipes and pumps that keep us going will help you better care for your future patients. Cardiovascular disease is the leading cause of death in the western world, and a common cause of hospital admission. I believe it to be the most fundamental medical specialty, and worthy of a detailed understanding wherever your future lies.

It was my aim that this book would save you from sleepless nights, headaches, panic attacks and frantic scrawling in lectures. I hope you find it a useful addition to your course notes, and I hope it saves you some of the most precious commodity around . . . time. I wish you all the very best of luck with your future studies.

Paul Sutton

The excellent Crash Course series summarizes the key learning points for the 'information overloaded' undergraduate medical student. The series format enhances learning through concise text, comprehension check boxes, and hints and tips boxes. The key salient points are presented in a user friendly and easy to read manner that enables the rapid assimilation of core knowledge.

The third edition of Crash Course: Cardiovascular System has been updated to provide contemporary emphasis on the cardiovascular system including current concepts of disease and emerging novel therapies. Complementary to the clinically orientated Crash Course: Cardiology, the book highlights all the essential basic knowledge that provides an invaluable foundation for application to clinical practice. The book takes the reader through first principles to inform the basis and presentation of cardiovascular disease, ultimately leading to the investigation and management of common cardiovascular disorders. This logical sequential progression enhances learning and understanding of the cardiovascular system in clinical medicine.

This book is a 'must' for the time pressed student who needs to use their revision time efficiently and effectively in the modern era of systems-based medical education.

David Newby
Faculty Advisor

More than a decade has now passed since work began on the first editions of the Crash Course series, and over four years since the publication of the second editions. Medicine never stands still, and the work of keeping this series relevant for today's students is an ongoing process. These third editions build upon the success of the preceding books and incorporate a great deal of new and revised material, keeping the series up to date with the latest medical research and developments in pharmacology and current best practice.

As always, we listen to feedback from the thousands of students who use Crash Course and have made further improvements to the layout and structure of the books. Each chapter now starts with a set of learning objectives, and the self-assessment sections have been enhanced and brought up to date with modern exam formats. We have also worked to integrate points of clinical relevance into the basic medical science material, which will not only add to the interest of the text but will reinforce the principles being described.

Despite fully revising the text, we hold fast to the principles on which we first developed the series: Crash Course will always bring you all the information you need to revise in compact, manageable volumes that integrate basic medical science and clinical practice. The books still maintain the balance between clarity and conciseness, and provide sufficient depth for those aiming at distinction. The authors are medical students and junior doctors who have recent experience of the exams you are now facing, and the accuracy of the material is checked by senior faculty members from across the UK.

I wish you all the best for your future careers!

Dr Dan Horton-Szar
Series Editor

Acknowledgements

I would like to thank Professor David Newby for his help, guidance and support and for telling me when I was wrong.

I would also like to thank Dr Lucy Smith for her contribution to the self-assessment section of the book.

Figure acknowledgements

Figs 2.16, 2.17 and 2.18 redrawn with permission from WJ Larsen. Human Embryology, 2nd edition. Churchill Livingstone, 1997

Fig. 2.24A redrawn with permission from PL Williams, ed. Gray's Anatomy, 37th edition. Churchill Livingstone, 1989

Fig. 2.24B redrawn with permission from A Davies, AGH Blakeley and C Kidd. Human Physiology. Churchill Livingstone, 2001

Fig. 2.37 redrawn with permission from CP Page, MJ Curtis, MC Sutter, MJA Walker, BB Hoffman, eds. Integrated Pharmacology. Mosby, 1997

Fig 2.40 redrawn with permission of the Physiological Society

Fig. 2.43 redrawn with permission from AC Guyton and JE Hall. Textbook of Medical Physiology, 9th edition. WB Saunders, 1995

Fig. 3.1 adapted with permission from Burton AC, Physiol Rev. 34: 619, 1954

Fig. 3.20 redrawn with permission from A Stevens and J Lowe. Human Histology, 2nd edition. Mosby, 1997

Fig. 3.23 adapted from Levick R. Introducing Cardiovascular Physiology. Butterworth–Heinemann, 1995. Reproduced by permission of Edward Arnold Ltd

Fig. 4.4 adapted from Levick R. Introducing Cardiovascular Physiology. Butterworth–Heinemann, 1995. Reproduced by permission of Edward Arnold Ltd

Fig. 5.2 redrawn with permission from Thelan IA, et al. Critical Care Nursing: Diagnosis and Management, 2nd edn. Mosby Year Book, 1994

Fig. 5.7 reproduced from Eur Heart J. Vol 17, March 1996. Courtesy of WB Saunders Co. Ltd

Figs 5.14–5.23 courtesy of T Lissauer and G Clayden. Illustrated Textbook of Paediatrics, 2nd edition. Mosby, 2001

Fig. 7.3 redrawn with permission from the Resuscitation Council of the United Kingdom (RCUK)

Fig. 9.3 redrawn with permission from O Epstein, D Perkin, D de Bono and J Cookson, eds. Clinical Examination, 2nd edition. Mosby International, 1997

Figs 9.13, 9.19–9.21, 9.24 and 9.25 courtesy of DE Newby and Neil R Grubb. Cardiology an Illustrated Colour Text, 1st edition. Elsevier, 2005

Figs 9.16 and 9.17 courtesy of Professor Dame M Turner-Warwick, Dr M Hodson, Professor B Corrin, and Dr I Kerr

Fig. 9.18 courtesy of Professor JJF Belch, Mr PT McCollum, Mr PA Stonebridge and Professor WF Walker

Figs 9.22, 9.23 and 9.26–9.30 courtesy of Dr A Timmis and Dr S Brecker

Dedication

To my mum, dad, sister and Lucy. Without your love and support I would not be where I am today.

Contents

Glossary

Afterload the resistance to the pressure and volume ejection from the heart.

Asystole absence of contraction. Asystole is when the heart has stopped beating and is different from ventricular fibrillation where the heart is still contracting, but not in a co-ordinated manner.

Bradycardia a heart rate <60 bpm.

Cardiac output (CO) the amount of blood pumped out by the heart every minute, calculated as stroke volume (SV) × heart rate (HR).

Central venous pressure (CVP) the pressure of blood in the great veins as they enter the right atrium.

Contractility the strength with which the myocardium contracts.

Diastole part of the cardiac cycle where the ventricles are relaxed and filling.

Ectopic an event occurring at a place other than its normal location, for example ventricular ectopics originate from the ventricles, not the sinoatrial node.

End-diastolic pressure (EDP) the amount of pressure in the ventricle at the end of diastole.

End-diastolic volume (EDV) the amount of blood in the ventricle at the end of diastole; the greatest amount found in the ventricle throughout the whole cardiac cycle.

Ejection fraction the proportion of EDV which is ejected by contraction.

Infarction tissue death caused by inadequate perfusion.

Laplace relationship a relationship between the tension, pressure and diameter of a container (implied blood vessel), as tension = diameter × pressure.

Mean arterial pressure (MAP) the average pressure in the system at any point in time, approximated as the diastolic pressure + (1/3 × pulse pressure).

Ohms Law a relationship between resistance, pressure and flow inside a container (implied blood vessel), as pressure = flow × resistance.

Perfusion movement of blood through an organ or tissue.

Preload the pressure and volume experienced by the heart before contraction.

Sinus rhythm a rhythm under direct control from the sinoatrial node.

Sphygmomanometer a device used for measuring blood pressure.

Starlings Law a phenomenon whereby the heart increases its output by increasing its strength of contraction when the fibres of the myocardium are stretched.

Stroke volume (SV) the amount of blood ejected from the left ventricle with each beat.

Stroke work (SW) the amount of external energy expended in one ventricular contraction. SW is the arterial pressure (AP) multiplied by the SV.

Syncope temporary loss of consciousness from reduced blood flow to the brain.

Systemic vascular resistance (SVR) the resistance to blood flow offered by all of the systemic vasculature, excluding the pulmonary vasculature. It is calculated as (MAP – right atrial pressure) / CO.

Systole part of the cardiac cycle where the ventricles are contracting.

Tachycardia a heart rate >100 bpm.

Total peripheral resistance (TPR) the resistance to the flow of blood in the whole system. It is calculated as arterial pressure / cardiac output.

BASIC MEDICAL SCIENCE

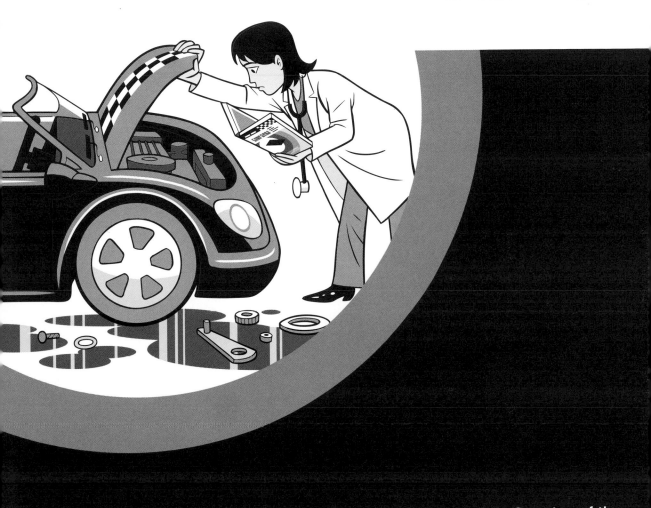

Overview of the cardiovascular system

WHY DO WE NEED A CARDIOVASCULAR SYSTEM?

The cardiovascular system serves to provide rapid transport of nutrients around the body and rapid removal of waste products. In smaller, less complex organisms than the human body there is no such system because their needs can be met by simple diffusion. Evolution of the cardiovascular system provided a means of aiding the diffusion process, allowing the development of larger organisms.

The cardiovascular system allows nutrients:

- To diffuse into the system at their source (e.g. oxygen from the lungs).
- To travel long distances quickly.
- To diffuse into tissues where they are needed (e.g. oxygen to working muscle).

This type of process is called convective transport, and is an active process (i.e. it requires energy). This energy is provided by the heart, with the vessels being the mode of convection.

The functions of the cardiovascular system rely on a medium for transport. This medium is blood, which is made up of cells (mainly red and white blood cells) and plasma (water, proteins, electrolytes etc.).

FUNCTIONS OF THE CARDIOVASCULAR SYSTEM

The main functions of the cardiovascular system are:

- Rapid transport of nutrients (oxygen, amino acids, glucose, fatty acids, water etc.).
- Removal of waste products of metabolism (carbon dioxide, urea, creatinine etc.).
- Hormonal control, by transporting hormones to their target organs and by secreting its own hormones (e.g. atrial natriuretic peptide).
- Temperature regulation, by controlling heat distribution between the body core and the skin.
- Reproduction, by producing erection of the penis and nutrition to the fetus via a complex system of placental blood flow.
- Host defence, transporting immune cells, antigen and other mediators (e.g. antibody).

THE HEART AND CIRCULATION

The heart is a double pump. It consists of two muscular pumps (the left and right ventricles). Each pump has its own reservoir (the left and right atrium).

The two pumps each serve a different circulation. Every blood cell flows first in one circulation and then moves into the other.

The right ventricle is the pump for the pulmonary circulation. It receives blood from the right atrium which is then pumped into the lungs through the pulmonary artery. Here it acquires oxygen and loses carbon dioxide; it then returns to the left atrium of the heart via the pulmonary veins and then enters the left ventricle.

The left ventricle is the pump for the systemic circulation. Blood is pumped from the left

3

ventricle to the rest of the body via the aorta. In the tissues of the body, nutrients and waste products are exchanged. Blood (which now carries less oxygen and more carbon dioxide) returns to the right atrium in the superior and inferior vena cavae and then re-enters the pulmonary circulation.

The pulmonary circulation is usually of lower pressure than the systemic circulation as the pulmonary vascular bed has a lower resistance.

The two circulations are operating simultaneously, with blood constantly flowing in each circulation. They can be thought of as being in series, with each circulation supplied by a different pump. This one-way, circular pathway for blood is brought about by the presence of valves in the heart and veins (Fig. 1.1).

The circulatory system is made up of arteries, veins, capillaries, and lymphatic vessels:

- Arteries transport blood from the heart to the body tissues.

- Capillaries are where diffusion of nutrients and waste products takes place.
- Veins return blood from the tissues to the heart.
- Lymphatic vessels return to the blood any excess water and nutrients that have diffused out of the capillaries.

Arteries carry oxygenated blood and veins carry deoxygenated blood. The two exceptions to this rule are the pulmonary and umbilical vessels (supplying the fetus) where this is reversed.

The amount of blood ejected from one ventricle during one minute is called the cardiac output. The cardiac output of each ventricle is equal overall, but there may be occasional beat-by-beat variation. The entire cardiac output of the right ventricle passes through the lungs. The cardiac output of the left ventricle passes into the aorta, and it is distributed to various organs and tissues according to their metabolic requirements or particular functions (e.g. the kidney receives 20% of cardiac output so that its excretory function can be maintained). This distribution can be changed to supply demand (e.g. during exercise, the flow to the skeletal muscle is increased considerably).

Blood is driven along the vessels by pressure. This pressure, which is produced by the ejection of blood from the ventricles, is highest in the aorta (about 120 mmHg above atmospheric pressure) and lowest in the great veins (almost atmospheric). It is this pressure difference that moves blood through the arterial tree, through the capillaries, and into the veins. In the veins, movement of blood is aided by one-way valves.

Arterial blood flow is pulsatile, with a higher pressure during systole (contraction) than during diastole (relaxation).

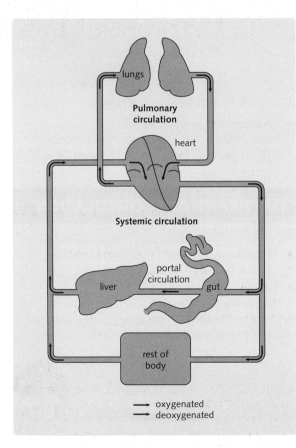

Fig. 1.1 Systemic and pulmonary circulations. Unidirectional flow is maintained by valves in the heart, pressure difference in the arterial tree, and valves in the venous system.

Systole is when the two ventricles contract simultaneously, whereas diastole is when the two ventricles relax together.

Structure and function of the heart

Objectives

You should be able to:

- Outline the anatomy of the heart, mediastinum and great vessels.
- Understand the embryological development of the cardiovascular system.
- Describe the heart skeleton and its function.
- State the different myocytes and know how they differ.
- Define the resting membrane potential and the factors that influence it.
- Sketch the action potential produced in the different cells of the myocardium, and explain the contribution of the different ion channels.
- Recall the cardiac cycle and explain how the jugular venous pressure, heart sounds and electrocardiogram relate to this.
- Sketch the conduction pathway.
- Define the terms cardiac output (CO), stroke volume (SV), stroke work (SW), heart rate (HR), end-diastolic volume (EDV), end-diastolic pressure (EDP), end-systolic pressure (ESP), end-systolic volume (ESV), central venous pressure (CVP), venous return (VR), total peripheral resistance (TPR), and contractility.
- State Starling's law of the heart and understand the physiological significance.

ORGANIZATION OF CARDIAC TISSUE

Anatomy of the heart and great vessels

Mediastinum

This is the space between the two lungs and pleurae. It contains all the structures of the chest except the lungs and pleurae (Figs 2.1 and 2.2).

The mediastinum extends from the superior thoracic aperture to the diaphragm and from the sternum to the vertebrae. The structures in the mediastinum are surrounded by loose connective tissue, nerves, blood, and lymph vessels. It can accommodate movement and volume changes.

The mediastinum is often subdivided into superior and inferior parts. The superior part contains:

- Anteriorly, the thymus.
- In the middle, the great vessels.
- Posteriorly, oesophagus, trachea, and thoracic duct.

Inferiorly, the mediastinum contains:

- Anteriorly, the thymus.
- In the middle, the heart and pericardium, great arteries, phrenic nerve, and main bronchi.
- Posteriorly, the oesophagus and thoracic aorta.

The heart is in the middle mediastinum, and it has the following relations:

- Superiorly, the great vessels and bronchi.
- Inferiorly, the diaphragm.
- Laterally, the pleurae and lungs.
- Anteriorly, the thymus.
- Posteriorly, the oesophagus.

The heart looks after itself first before 'feeding' other organs. The coronary arteries are the first branches of the ascending aorta, and fill mainly during diastole as the myocardium relaxes.

Pericardium

The pericardium is a fibroserous sac which consists of tough fibrous tissue enclosing the heart. The outer surface of the heart and the inner surface of pericardium are covered with transparent layers of serous pericardium. Between these layers, there is pericardial fluid.

The base of the pericardium is fused with the central tendon of the diaphragm. The pericardium is also fused with the tunica adventitia of the great vessels entering and leaving the heart. Anteriorly, the pericardium is joined to the sternum by the sternopericardial ligaments.

There are two sinuses (pouches or pockets) in the pericardium; they are formed by the folding of the embryological heart, which produces reflections in the pericardium:

- The transverse pericardial sinus is a recess within the pericardium, posterior to the aorta and pulmonary trunk and anterior to the superior vena cava.
- The oblique pericardial sinus is a blind recess formed by the inferior vena cava and pulmonary veins.

External structure of the heart

The heart lies obliquely about two-thirds to the left and one-third to the right of the median plane (Figs 2.3–2.5). It has the following surfaces:

- The base of the heart is located posteriorly and formed mainly by the left atrium.
- The apex of the heart is formed by the left ventricle and is posterior to the 5th intercostal space.
- The sternocostal surface of the heart is formed mainly by the right ventricle.
- The diaphragmatic surface is formed mainly by the left ventricle and part of the right ventricle.
- The pulmonary surface is mainly formed by the left ventricle.

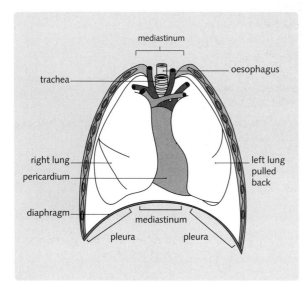

Fig. 2.1 Anterior view of the mediastinum.

Fig. 2.2 Lateral view of the mediastinum.

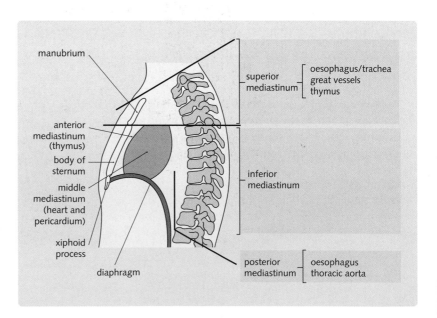

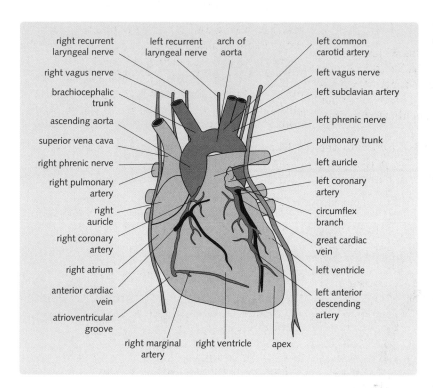

Fig. 2.3 Sternocostal external view of the heart.

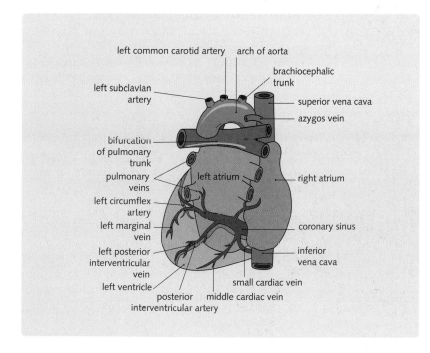

Fig. 2.4 Postero-inferior external view of the heart.

Fig. 2.5 Surface markings of the heart (a, aortic valve; m, mitral valve; p, pulmonary valve; t, tricuspid valve). These are anatomical relations – see Chapter 8 for auscultatory areas.

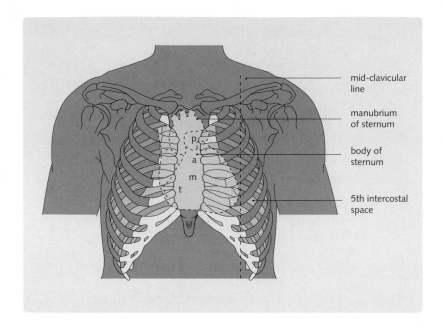

mid-clavicular line

manubrium of sternum

body of sternum

5th intercostal space

The heart borders of the anterior surface are as follows:

- Right: right atrium.
- Left: left ventricle and left auricle.
- Inferior: right ventricle mainly and part of left ventricle.
- Superior: right and left auricles.

Internal structure of the heart

The internal structure of the heart is shown in Fig. 2.6. The right atrium contains the orifices of the superior and inferior venae cavae and coronary sinus.

The right ventricle is separated from the right atrium by the tricuspid (three cusps) valve. The right ventricle is separated from its outflow tract (the pulmonary trunk) by the pulmonary valve. This has three semilunar valve cusps.

The left atrium has the orifices of four pulmonary veins in its posterior wall. The left atrium is separated from the left ventricle by the mitral (sometimes referred to as bicuspid, i.e. two cusps) valve. The left ventricle is separated from its outflow tract (the aorta) by the aortic valve. This also has three semilunar valve cusps.

Coronary arteries

The coronary arteries are shown in Figs 2.7 and 2.8. The left coronary artery arises from the left anterior cusp of the aortic valve. The right coronary artery arises from the right anterior aortic sinus just above the right anterior cusp of the aortic valve. The coronary arteries are the first branches of the aorta; the heart supplies itself with a blood supply before any other organ.

Knowledge of the arterial supply to the myocardium is essential in determining which vessel is affected in ischaemic heart disease, and allows us to predict the sequelae of an event. Inferior infarcts caused by disease of the right coronary artery, for example, are more prone to bradyarrhythmias as this artery also supplies the sinoatrial and atrioventricular nodes.

Coronary veins

The coronary veins drain mainly into the coronary sinus, which drains directly into the right atrium (Figs 2.9 and 2.10). There are some small veins that drain directly into the heart chambers. Generally, these drain into the right side of the heart.

Great vessels

The 'great vessels' is the term used to denote the large arteries and veins that are directly related to

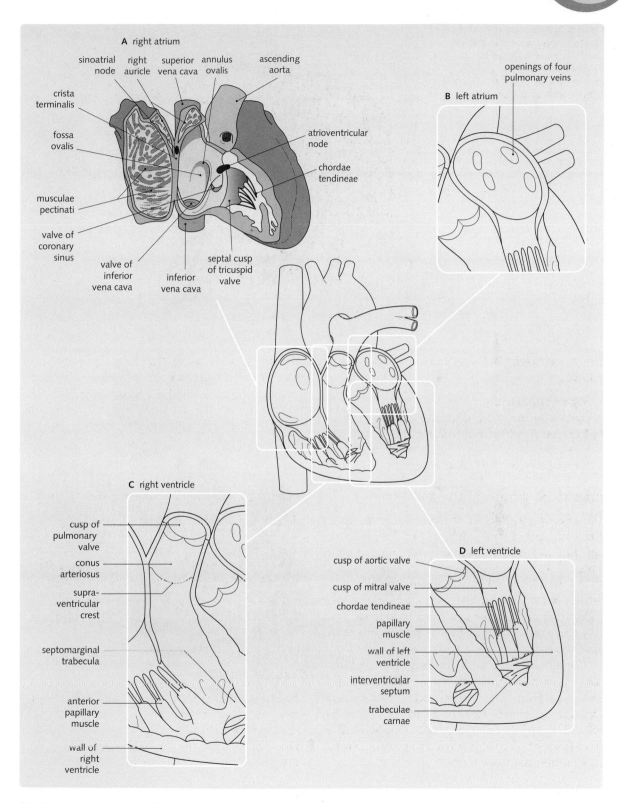

Fig. 2.6 Internal structure of the four chambers of the heart. (A) Right atrium. (B) Left atrium. (C) Right ventricle. (D) Left ventricle.

Fig. 2.7 Anterior surface of the heart showing coronary arteries. The left coronary artery has two terminal branches: the anterior interventricular branch (also called the left anterior descending or Widow's artery) and the circumflex branch. The anterior interventricular branch supplies both ventricles and the interventricular septum. The circumflex branch supplies the left atrium and the inferior part of the left ventricle. The right coronary artery supplies the sinoatrial (SA) node via the right atrial branch.

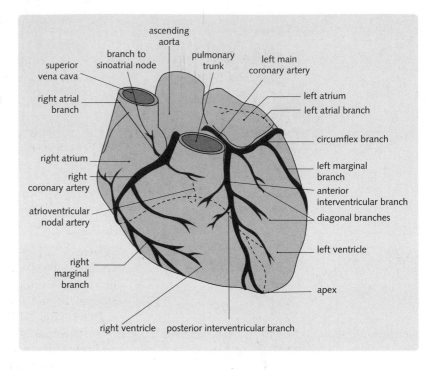

Fig. 2.8 Postero-inferior surface of the heart showing coronary arteries. The right coronary artery gives off a right marginal branch (see Fig. 2.7) and a large posterior interventricular branch. Near the apex, the posterior interventricular branch may anastomose with the anterior interventricular branch of the left coronary artery. The right coronary artery mainly supplies the right atrium, right ventricle, and interventricular septum. It may also supply part of the left atrium and left ventricle. The nodal branch supplies the atrioventricular (AV) node.

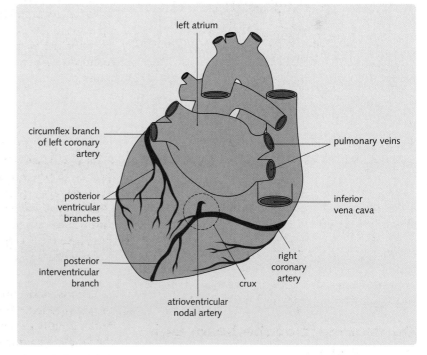

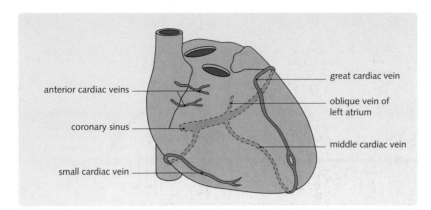

Fig. 2.9 Anterior view of the heart showing coronary veins.

anterior cardiac veins

coronary sinus

small cardiac vein

great cardiac vein

oblique vein of left atrium

middle cardiac vein

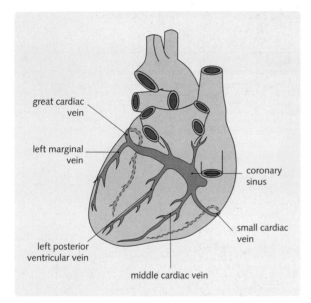

great cardiac vein

left marginal vein

left posterior ventricular vein

middle cardiac vein

coronary sinus

small cardiac vein

Fig. 2.10 Postero-inferior view of the heart showing coronary veins.

the heart. The great arteries include the pulmonary trunk and the aorta (and sometimes its three main branches: the brachiocephalic, the left common carotid, and the left subclavian). The great veins include the pulmonary veins and the superior and inferior venae cavae. The great vessels and their thoracic branches are illustrated in Figs 2.11–2.13.

Development of the heart and great vessels

The heart develops in the cardiogenic region of the mesoderm in week 3. This region is at the cranial end of the embryonic disc. Angioblastic cords

(aggregates of endothelial cell precursors) develop and here they coalesce to form two lateral endocardial tubes. During week 4, these tubes fuse together to form the primitive heart tube and the heart begins to pump (Fig. 2.14).

From weeks 5 to 8, the primitive heart tube folds and remodels to form the four-chambered heart. Initially, the primitive heart tube develops a series of expansions separated by shallow sulci (infoldings, Fig. 2.15).

The primitive atrium will give rise to parts of both future atria. The primitive ventricle will make up most of the left ventricle. The bulbus cordis will form the right ventricle. The truncus arteriosus will form the ascending aorta and the pulmonary trunk.

There are many difficult terms in embryology. Try to understand them by considering what process the term describes. For example, the septum primum is the first (primus means first in Latin) septum to form and septum secundum is the second septum to form.

Venous blood initially enters the sinus horns of the sinus venosus from the cardinal veins (a branch of the umbilical vein). Within the next few weeks, the whole systemic venous return is shifted to the right sinus horn through the newly formed superior and inferior venae cavae. The left sinus horn becomes the coronary sinus, which drains the myocardium.

Fig. 2.11 The thoracic aorta and its branches.

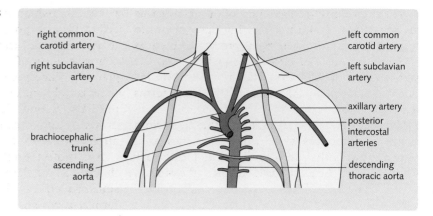

Fig. 2.12 Veins of the thorax.

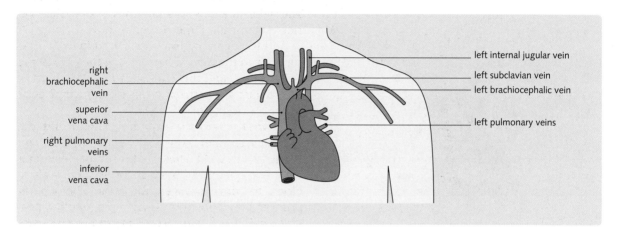

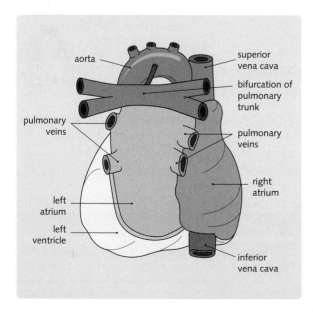

Fig. 2.13 Posterior view of the pulmonary vessels.

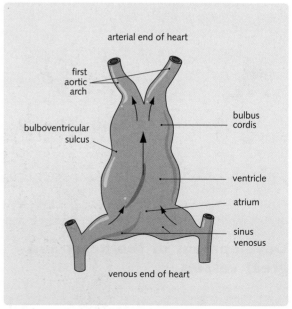

Fig. 2.14 Primitive heart tube at 21 days.

The right sinus horn and part of the venae cavae are incorporated into the growing right atrium to form the posterior wall by a process known as intussusception (Fig. 2.16). This gives rise to the smooth wall of the bulk of the atrium, while the original, trabeculated right half of the atrium forms the right auricle.

The original left half of the primitive atrium grows a pulmonary vein, which branches as it moves towards the lungs to form the pulmonary venous system. Eventually, the trunk of the pulmo-nary vein (which has grown from the primitive atrium) is incorporated (again by intussusception) to form most of the left atrium. As this process continues more of the pulmonary venous system is gradually incorporated into the atrium. Initially there is only one orifice, but the process continues until the second bifurcation is reached and four orifices result. Again, the original, trabeculated atrial wall forms the left auricle.

A pair of valves (the venous valves) develops at the orifices of the venae cavae and the coronary sinus. Superior to these orifices, the valves fuse to form a transient septum spurium. The left valve eventually becomes part of the septum secundum. The right valve develops into the valves of the inferior vena cava and the coronary sinus.

A ridge of tissue, the crista terminalis, forms superior to the right valve marking the edge of the right auricle, and this will eventually form part of the conduction pathway from the sinoatrial node to the atrioventricular node.

In weeks 5–6, the septum primum and the septum secundum grow to separate the right and left atria (Fig. 2.17). These septa are incomplete and leave two openings (foramina or ostia) that allow blood to move between the atria. The septum primum grows downwards from the superior, posterior wall. The foramen (ostium primum) it creates narrows as the septum grows.

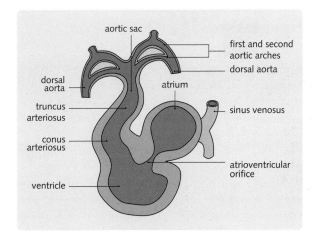

Fig. 2.15 Primitive heart tube as it folds and expands.

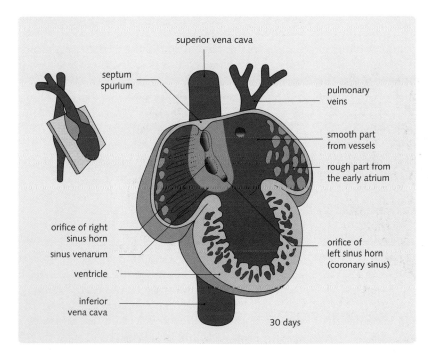

30 days

Fig. 2.16 Initial differentiation of the primitive atrium. The primitive atrium derives from two tissues: the rough part from early atrial tissue; the smooth part from venous tissue that spreads as the veins 'push' into the developing atrium. (Redrawn with permission from Larsen W J. Human embryology, 2nd edn. Edinburgh: Churchill Livingstone, 1997.)

Fig. 2.17 Initial septation of the atria. The septum primum forms at day 33, and eventually leaves a hole (the ostium secundum). The septum secundum develops later at day 40 and is deficient at the foramen ovale. (Redrawn with permission from Larsen W J. Human embryology, 2nd edn. Edinburgh: Churchill Livingstone, 1997.)

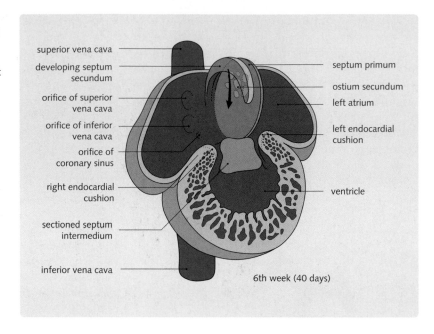

superior vena cava

developing septum secundum

orifice of superior vena cava

orifice of inferior vena cava

orifice of coronary sinus

right endocardial cushion

sectioned septum intermedium

inferior vena cava

septum primum

ostium secundum

left atrium

left endocardial cushion

ventricle

6th week (40 days)

The endocardium around the atrioventricular canal (between the atria and the ventricles) grows to form four expansions. These are the left, right, superior, and inferior endocardial cushions.

At the end of week 6, the superior and inferior cushions meet and fuse together to form the septum intermedium creating the left and right atrioventricular canals. At the same time, the edge of the septum primum fuses with the septum intermedium, closing the ostium primum. However, before complete closure of the ostium primum, cell death in the superior part of the septum primum creates small openings, which join together to form the ostium secundum. This maintains the shunt between the two atria.

While the septum primum is growing, a thicker septum secundum also starts to form. This septum secundum does not meet the septum intermedium, leaving an opening called the foramen ovale near the floor of the right atrium.

Blood now has to shunt from the right to the left atrium through the two staggered openings in the septum, the foramen ovale and the ostium secundum (Fig. 2.18). At birth, the two septa are fused together to abolish any foramen between the two atria.

During weeks 5–6 the atrioventricular valves develop. The heart undergoes some changes that bring the atria and ventricles into their correct positions and align the outflow tracks with the ventricles.

The inferior part of the bulboventricular sulcus grows into the muscular ventricular septum. Growth stops in week 7 to wait for the left outflow track to develop, leaving an interventricular foramen.

In weeks 7–8 the truncus arteriosus (the common outflow tract of the heart) is divided in two by a spiral process of central septation, which results in the formation of the aorta and pulmonary trunk. This septum is called the truncoconal septum.

This septum also grows into the ventricles, and it forms the membranous ventricular septum, which joins the muscular ventricular septum. This completes the septation of the ventricles.

Swellings develop at the inferior end of the truncus arteriosus, and these give rise to the semilunar arterial valves.

Congenital abnormalities

The embryological development of the heart is a complex process involving many coordinated steps. Defects arise if the process does not occur correctly. Congenital cardiovascular abnormalities are the most common congenital defects in live births. The most common abnormalities include:

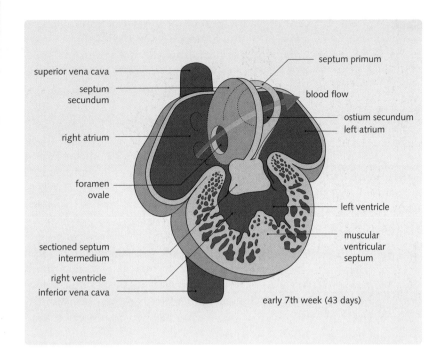

superior vena cava

septum secundum

right atrium

foramen ovale

sectioned septum intermedium

right ventricle
inferior vena cava

septum primum

blood flow

ostium secundum
left atrium

left ventricle

muscular ventricular septum

early 7th week (43 days)

Fig. 2.18 Completed septation of the atria. The septum primum is deficient superiorly at the ostium secundum. The septum secundum is deficient inferiorly at the foramen ovale. Blood shunts from the right atrium through these two holes in the septa to the left atrium. In this way, blood bypasses the lungs in the fetal circulation. As these two openings are staggered, fusion of the septum primum and secundum will abolish any shunt between the atria. (Redrawn with permission from Larsen W J. Human embryology, 2nd edn. Edinburgh: Churchill Livingstone, 1997.)

- Bicuspid aortic valve.
- Coarctation (narrowing) of the aorta.
- Ventricular septal defect (VSD).
- Atrial septal defect (ASD).
- Atrioventricular septal defect (AVSD).
- Tricuspid and mitral valve defects.
- Persistent truncus arteriosus.
- Transposition of the great arteries (TGA).
- Tetralogy of Fallot.

VSD can result from failure of the muscular and membranous septa to fuse, failure of the endocardial cushions to fuse (also causes AVSD), or perforation of the muscular septum during development.

There are many types of ASD, including patent foramen ovale and secundum ASD. Patent foramen ovale occurs when the septum primum and septum secundum fail to fuse together at birth, allowing blood to shunt across. A secundum ASD results when the septum secundum fails to grow completely and so does not cover the ostium secundum. When the septum primum and secundum fuse a hole is still present.

AVSD can result from failure of the superior and inferior endocardial cushions to fuse, and is associated exclusively with Down syndrome.

Tricuspid and mitral valve defects result from errors in the development of the valves from the ventricular wall.

In persistent truncus arteriosus, the truncoconal septum fails to form, leading to a common outflow tract for both ventricles. There is also a VSD.

TGA occurs when the truncoconal septum develops, but it does not spiral. The left ventricle pumps blood into the pulmonary trunk and the right ventricle pumps blood into the aorta. There is also a patent foramen ovale or patent ductus arteriosus to allow blood to mix.

Tetralogy of Fallot is a combination of pulmonary stenosis, right ventricular hypertrophy, overriding aorta, and VSD. The primary problem is failure of the outflow regions to align properly. This causes stenosis around the subpulmonary outlet, which leads to right ventricular hypertrophy. A VSD also occurs because of malalignment, as fusion between the membranous and muscular septum cannot take place. The abnormality also displaces the aorta to the right causing it to be overriding.

These congenital abnormalities are illustrated and further discussed in Chapter 5.

Tissue layers of the heart and pericardium

The heart contains three layers:

- Pericardium.
- Myocardium.
- Endocardium (Fig. 2.19).

Pericardium

The pericardium consists of an outer fibrous pericardial sac, enclosing the whole heart, and an inner double layer of flat mesothelial cells, called the serous pericardium. The two layers of the serous pericardium are:

- The parietal pericardium, which is attached to the fibrous sac.
- The visceral pericardium (or epicardium), which covers the heart's outer surface.

The serous pericardium produces approximately 50 mL of pericardial fluid, which sits in the peri-cardial cavity formed by the parietal and visceral layers. This fluid is mainly for lubrication.

The epicardium's thin internal layer of connective tissue contains adipose tissue, nerves, and the coronary arteries and veins.

Myocardium

Myocardium is the thickest layer of the heart, and it consists of cardiac muscle cells. The thickness and cell diameter are greatest in the left ventricle and thinnest in the atria. All the muscle layers attach to the heart skeleton, which provides a base for contraction.

The atrial myocardium secretes atrial natriuretic peptide (ANP) when stretched, promoting salt and water excretion. The ventricular myocardium however secretes brain natriuretic peptide (BNP) when stretched. Whilst this is rather a misnomer, it is increasingly being used to monitor left ventricular dysfunction.

> When examining the cardiovascular system it is important to remember that the right ventricle lies anteriorly and faces the sternocostal surface. In certain conditions causing pulmonary hypertension, the right ventricle is forced to work excessively hard, and this can be felt as a heave on the precordium.

Endocardium

The endocardium has three layers: an outermost connective tissue layer (which contains nerves, veins and Purkinje fibres), a middle layer of connective tissue, and an inner endothelium of flat endothelial cells.

Heart skeleton

The heart skeleton consists of fibrotendinous (fibrocollagenous) rings of dense connective tissue that encircle the base of the aorta and pulmonary trunk and the atrioventricular openings (Fig. 2.20). The heart valves and cardiac muscle attach to these rings. The heart skeleton forms the base of the heart for contraction.

The skeleton also electrically insulates the atria from the ventricles. The membranous interventricular septum is a downwards extension of the fibro-

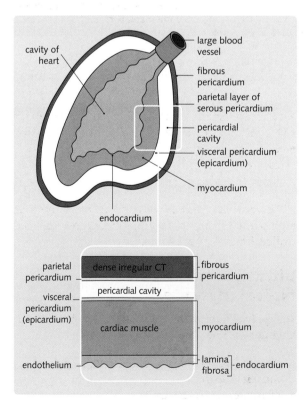

Fig. 2.19 Tissue layers of the heart and pericardium (CT, connective tissue).

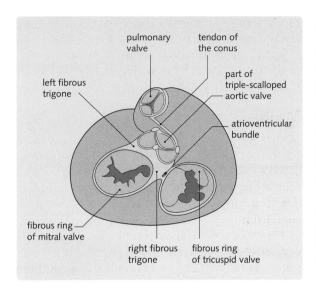

Fig. 2.20 Superior view of the heart skeleton. Vessels and external muscle layers have been removed.

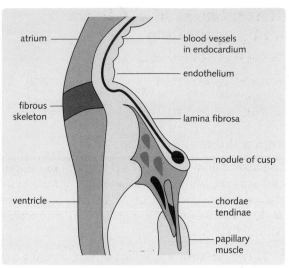

Fig. 2.21 Structure of a heart valve.

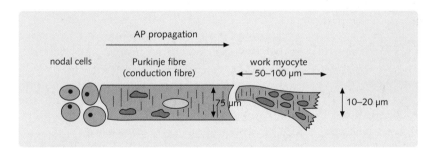

Fig. 2.22 Types of myocytes. The action potential (AP) is initiated in the nodal cells. It is then rapidly conducted through the Purkinje fibres to the work myocytes where contraction occurs.

collagenous tissue, and it contains the bundle of His. The atrioventricular node and the bundle of His form the only conduction pathway through the skeleton and, therefore, the only electrical link between the atria and the ventricles.

Valves

The heart valves are avascular (i.e. they have no blood supply) (Fig. 2.21). This is important if bacteria invade the valves, because there is little immune reaction and infective endocarditis may result.

CELLULAR PHYSIOLOGY OF THE HEART

Cardiac myocytes

There are three types of myocytes – work myocytes, nodal cells, and conduction fibres (Fig. 2.22):

- Work myocytes are the main contractile cells.
- Nodal cells generate cardiac electrical impulses.
- Conduction (Purkinje) fibres allow fast conduction of action potentials around the heart (see also p. 19).

The myocardium is innervated by autonomic (sympathetic and parasympathetic) nerves controlled from the brainstem.

Ultrastructure of the typical myocyte

The typical cardiac myocyte (Fig. 2.23) has the following features:

- Length of 50–100 μm (shorter than skeletal muscle fibres).
- Diameter of 10–20 μm.
- Single, central nucleus.
- Branched structure.

Fig. 2.23 Cardiac myocyte arrangement. Myocytes are branched, and they attach to each other through desmosomes to form muscle fibres. Gap junctions enable rapid electrical conductivity between cells. There is an extensive sarcoplasmic reticulum, which is the internal Ca²⁺ store. The contractile elements within each cell produce characteristic bands and lines. In between each myofibril unit there are rows of mitochondria. Accompanying blood vessels and connective tissue lie alongside each muscle fibre. (Redrawn with permission from Tortora G J, Grabowski S R. Principles of anatomy and physiology, 9th edn. New York: John Wiley & Sons, 2000.)

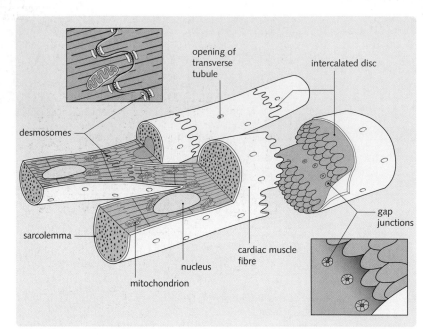

- Attached to neighbouring cells via intercalated disks at the branch points. These cell junctions consist of desmosomes (which hold the cells together via proteoglycan bridges) and gap junctions (which allow electrical conductivity).
- Many mitochondria arranged in rows between the intracellular myofibrils.
- T (transverse) tubules organized in diads with cisternae of sarcoplasmic reticulum (Fig. 2.24), which enable rapid electrical conduction deep into the cell, activating the whole contractile apparatus.
- Extensive sarcoplasmic reticulum, which stores Ca²⁺ ions necessary for electrical activity and contraction.

Each myocyte contains many myofibril-like units (similar to the myofibrils of skeletal muscle) (Fig. 2.24). These myofibril-like units are made up of many sarcomeres attached end-to-end and collected into a bundle.

A sarcomere is the basic contractile unit. It is composed of two bands, the A band and the I band, between two Z lines.

The A (anisotropic) band is made up of thick myosin filaments and some interdigitating actin filaments.

The I (isotropic) band is made up of thin actin filaments that do not overlap with myosin fila-ments. Troponin and tropomyosin are also con-tained in the thin filaments.

The Z line is a dark-staining structure containing α-actinin protein that provides attachment for the thin filaments.

Excitation and action potentials

Resting membrane potential

The resting membrane potential of a cardiac cell is approximately −80 mV (Fig. 2.25). This value is determined by the distribution of ions across the membrane, and the differential permeability of the membrane. In cardiac myocytes it is the K⁺ gradient that is the major determinant of the resting mem-brane potential. The potential can be predicted using the Nernst equation:

$$E_K = -65 \log ([K^+]_{out}/[K^+]_{in})$$

There is a discrepancy between the predicted value and the actual value. This is due to the leakage of small numbers of Na⁺ ions inward and K⁺ ions outward across the membrane and the action of the enzyme Na⁺/K⁺ ATPase, which acts to preserve the resting potential.

Digitalis (digoxin) inhibits the sodium pump, partially lowering the transmembrane Na⁺ gradi-ent (see Chapter 5).

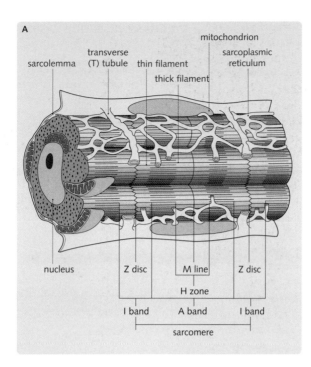

Fig. 2.24 Electronmicrographic appearance of cardiac muscle. (A) Each myocyte has rows of mitochondria in between myofibril-like units. There is also an extensive sarcoplasmic reticulum and T tubule system. (B) Close-up of a myofibril-like unit shows the following bands: A band, myosin with some actin; I band, actin; Z line, attachment point for actin. (Reproduced with permission from [A] Williams P L (ed). Gray's anatomy, 37th edn. Edinburgh: Churchill Livingstone, 1989; [B] Davies A, Blakeley A G H, Kidd C. Human physiology. Edinburgh: Churchill Livingstone, 2001.)

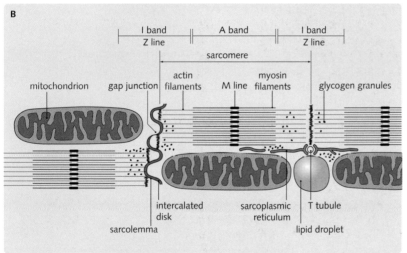

Ion concentrations			
Ion	Extracellular concentration (mmol/L)	Intracellular concentration (mmol/L)	Equilibrium potential (mV)
Na$^+$	145	10	70
K$^+$	4	135	−94
Cl$^-$	120	30	−36

Fig. 2.25 Intracellular and extracellular ionic concentrations.

Action potential

Understanding cardiac action potentials and how these relate to ion changes and ventricular filling is a very common exam question.

The cardiac action potential (Fig. 2.26) lasts about 300 ms in work myocytes. The arrival of an action potential from a neighbouring cell causes the cell membrane to depolarize and opens Na^+ channels, generating the fast upstroke. This subsequently opens Ca^{2+} channels and this produces the plateau phase. K^+ channels are also opened and this eventually leads to repolarization. The late part of the plateau phase is sustained by the action of the Na^+–Ca^{2+} exchanger. Nerve action potentials, in contrast to the cardiac action potential, last only 3 ms, and they do not have a plateau phase.

The plateau phase, caused by the influx of Ca^{2+}, determines the strength of contraction and it makes the cardiac cell refractory for the duration of the twitch, preventing tetanic contractions.

Na^+ channels are blocked by tetrodotoxin, leading to a slower upstroke and action potential.

Ca^{2+} channels are blocked by a group of drugs called Ca^{2+} channel blockers (e.g. verapamil), leading to shorter plateau phase and action potential, which weakens contraction. They are opened by adrenaline, enhancing the plateau phase and increasing contraction.

K^+ channels are blocked by caesium, leading to prolonged repolarization.

Variation in action potential

Sinoatrial node

The sinoatrial (SA) node is located in the posterior wall of the right atrium. It is the cardiac pacemaker and is responsible for initiating the depolarization and, therefore, contraction of the whole heart.

The SA node's resting membrane potential is unstable and so when it reaches a threshold value it triggers off an action potential (Fig. 2.27). The upstroke of the action potential is slow because it is mediated by a Ca^{2+} current and not a Na^+ current, as in the fast upstrokes of ventricular myocytes.

The SA node is controlled by the autonomic nervous system. Sympathetic stimulation increases the rate of decay of the resting membrane potential and, therefore, it causes more frequent action potentials. Parasympathetic stimulation has the opposite effect.

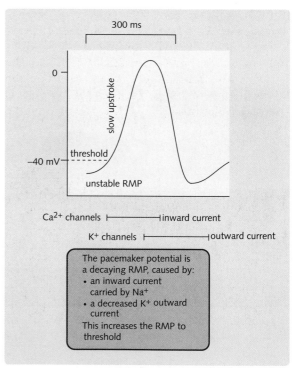

Fig. 2.27 The sinoatrial (SA) node action potential and the generation of the natural pacemaker potential. Voltage-gated calcium channels open once the resting membrane potential (RMP) has decayed above threshold.

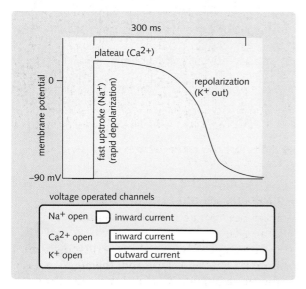

Fig. 2.26 Diagram of cardiac action potential showing the timing of ionic current flow.

A chronotropic agent is one that increases (positive chronotrope) or decreases (negative chronotrope) the heart rate. An inotropic agent is one that increases (positive inotrope) or decreases (negative inotrope) the force of contraction. The action potential varies in different myocytes. Fig. 2.28 shows the action potentials through the conduction pathway.

Excitation–contraction coupling

Contraction of cardiac muscle occurs in a similar manner to that of skeletal muscle.

Active myosins project from the thick filaments (also composed of myosins) and when activated by Ca^{2+} and adenosine triphosphate (ATP), they pull the thin filaments (actin) together to cause shortening. This process involves troponin C and tropomyosin. Full details of this can be found in the title *Crash Course: Musculoskeletal System*.

Contraction is initiated by a rise in cytoplasmic Ca^{2+} as the contractile proteins are dependent upon Ca^{2+} (Fig. 2.29). Relaxation is brought about by a decrease in intracellular Ca^{2+} concentration (written $[Ca^{2+}]$) (Fig. 2.30), and so the duration of contraction is determined by the duration of the plateau. The force of contraction is directly related to $[Ca^{2+}]$ and contractile protein sensitivity to Ca^{2+}. The sensitivity of these proteins is increased by the initial stretch of the sarcomere. Contraction is also dependent on ATP, which is supplied by the mitochondria.

Calcium is the key ion in muscles. Changing its concentration is the basis of most of the actions of the nervous system, hormones, and some drugs that act on the heart and vessels (e.g. noradrenaline from sympathetic nerves increases intracellular Ca^{2+} and increases contraction).

Effect of inotropic agents

Inotropic agents increase force of contractility by affecting cytoplasmic (intracellular) Ca^{2+}. They increase cytoplasmic Ca^{2+} by:

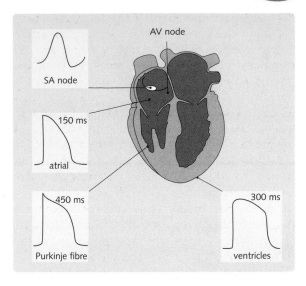

Fig. 2.28 Action potentials in different cardiac myocytes (SA, sinoatrial).

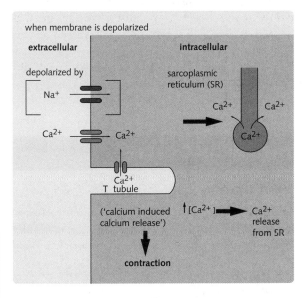

Fig. 2.29 Excitation and its effect on the myocyte (SR, sarcoplasmic reticulum).

- Increasing Ca^{2+} influx – noradrenaline increases Ca^{2+} entry by opening more Ca^{2+} channels.
- Decreasing Ca^{2+} removal – digitalis (digoxin) inhibits Na^+/K^+ ATPase and, therefore, reduces the Na^+ gradient. This, in turn, reduces the action of the Na^+–Ca^{2+} exchanger. This decreases Ca^{2+} removal from the cell.

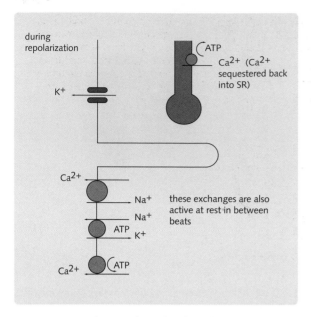

Fig. 2.30 Ion exchanges that take place during relaxation (SR, sarcoplasmic reticulum).

Increased heart rate lessens the resting time that the cell has between beats. This also decreases Ca^{2+} removal, causing a gradual increase in cytoplasmic Ca^{2+} and, therefore, force. This is called the staircase or Treppe effect.

THE CARDIAC CYCLE

Definition

The cardiac cycle (Fig. 2.31) is the sequence of pressure and volume changes that takes place during cardiac activity (Figs 2.32 and 2.33). A cycle time of 0.9 s is taken at rest.

Events of the cardiac cycle

Ventricular filling (diastole)

The atria and ventricles are all relaxed initially, and there is passive filling of the ventricles. The volume increases until a neutral ventricular volume is reached. Further filling, driven by venous pressure, causes the ventricle to distend. This causes ventricular pressure to rise. Contraction of the atria further increases the filling of the ventricles. However, this accounts for only about 15–20% of ventricular filling at rest. The volume now in the ventricle is termed the end-diastolic volume.

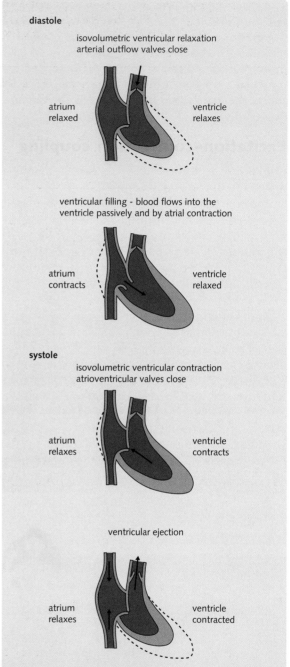

Fig. 2.31 The cardiac cycle.

Isovolumetric contraction (systole)

The contraction of the ventricles increases ventricular pressure. Ventricular pressure rises above atrial pressure, thereby closing the atrioventricular valves. This creates a closed chamber. As ventricular

The cardiac cycle				
	Diastole	**Systole**		**Diastole**
Stage	Ventricular filling	Isovolumetric contraction	Ejection	Isovolumetric relaxation
Duration (s)	0.5	0.05	0.3	0.08
AV valves	Open	Closed	Closed	Closed
Arterial valves	Closed	Closed	Open	Closed
Ventricular pressure	Falls then slowly rises	Rapid rise	Rises then slowly falls	Rapid fall
Ventricular volume	Increases	Constant	Decreases	Constant

Fig. 2.32 Summary table of the stages of the cardiac cycle. Changes at fixed volume are referred to as isovolumetric, and precede the later contraction or dilation of the ventricles (AV, atrioventricular).

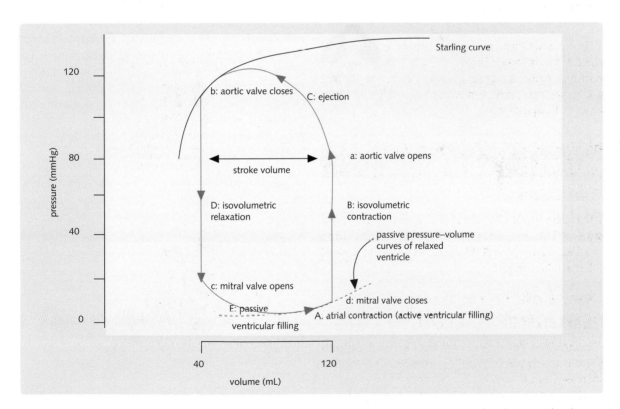

Fig. 2.33 Pressure–volume cycle of left ventricle. The most significant pressure changes occur within the ventricles during the isovolumetric stages.

contraction proceeds, wall tension increases, causing a rapid rise in ventricular pressure. The rate of rise of pressure is a measure of cardiac contractility.

Ejection (systole)

Ventricular pressure rises above arterial pressure, opening the arterial valves. This causes a rapid initial rise in arterial pressure, and then the pressure starts to fall as contraction fades.

The momentum of blood prevents immediate valve closure, even when ventricular pressure falls below arterial pressure. Eventually, the arterial valves close, which creates the brief rise in arterial pressure called the dicrotic wave notch.

The ventricle does not empty completely. There is an end-systolic volume of about 50% of end-diastolic volume, which can be used to increase stroke volume when necessary.

Venous return = Right heart input & output = Pulmonary blood flow = Left heart input & output = Systemic blood flow – BECAUSE THEY ARE ALL IN SERIES!

Isovolumetric relaxation (diastole)

The closure of both sets of valves creates an enclosed chamber. The relaxation of sarcomeres plus collagen recoil drops the ventricular pressure. When ventricular pressure falls below atrial pressure, the atrioventricular valves open leading to filling.

Cardiac cycle and normal heart sounds

Four heart sounds can be differentiated (Fig. 2.34):

- First – due to mitral and tricuspid valve closure (the atrioventricular valves).
- Second – due to aortic and pulmonary valve closure (the semilunar/arterial valves).
- Third – due to the sudden rapid flow of blood into the ventricles in diastole.
- Fourth – due to flow of blood into the ventricles due to atrial systole (contraction).

Usually only the first and second heart sounds are audible as a 'lubb-dupp' every beat.

The second heart sound can be split, appearing to be two different distinguishable sounds. This is caused by inspiration increasing right ventricular filling and, therefore, increasing the time taken for right ventricular ejection and delaying pulmonary valve closure. Left ventricular ejection time is shortened leading to faster closure of the aortic valve. This is termed physiological splitting, and it is normal.

Valvular abnormalities (stenosis and incompetence) lead to murmurs, with turbulent blood flow causing extra sounds. These are discussed more fully in Chapter 9.

Fig. 2.34 Displayed at the top of the diagram is pressure and outflow in left side of heart. Pressure in the left ventricle increases slightly during left atrial contraction (A). The most rapid increase in pressure occurs during isovolumetric contraction (B). The increase in pressure caused by ventricular contraction closes the mitral valve (a). When left ventricular pressure just exceeds aortic pressure the aortic valve opens (b) leading to ejection (C). Pressure rises to a peak and then falls, leading to aortic valve closure (c). Isovolumetric relaxation then occurs (D) and eventually left ventricular pressure is just below left atrial pressure, leading to the opening of the mitral valve (d). This allows passive filling of the ventricles (E). Below this the normal electrocardiogram is displayed as it relates to the cardiac cycle (see p. 22). The jugular venous pressure (JVP) (shown below) reflects right atrial pressure due to the close proximity of the central veins to the right atrium and its activity (a_2, atrial contraction; c_2, movement of the tricuspid valve ring into the atrium when the ventricle contracts – in the jugular vein this may also be due to movement of the carotid artery in systole; v, peak pressure in the atrium due to atrial filling – the tricuspid valve is just about to open; x, x descent due to atrial relaxation; y, y descent due to ventricular filling). Finally, the heart sounds are displayed (S_1, closure of the mitral and tricuspid valves 'lubb'; S_2, closure of the aortic and pulmonary valves 'dupp'; S_3, passive ventricular filling – a low frequency sound; S_4, active ventricular filling due to atrial contraction – a low frequency sound).

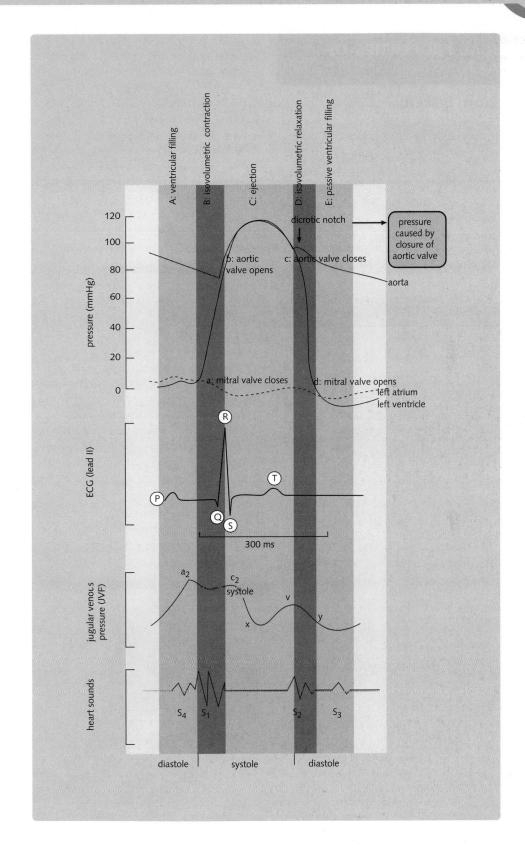

ELECTRICAL PROPERTIES OF THE HEART

Conduction system

The aim of the conduction system (Figs 2.35 and 2.36) is to allow atrial and ventricular contraction to be coordinated for maximum efficiency.

The steps of depolarization of the heart are as follows:

1. Depolarization is initiated in the SA node (see p. 20).
2. Depolarization spreads through adjacent atrial work cells causing atrial systole in both atria.

Fibre size diameter and conduction velocity		
Muscle cell (myocyte)	Diameter (mm)	Conduction velocity (m/s)
Atrial work cell	10	1
AV node	3	0.05
Purkinje fibres	75	4
Ventricular work cell	10–20	1

Fig. 2.35 Fibre diameter and conduction velocity of the different cardiac cells.

3. At the AV node (the beginning of the only electrical pathway through the fibrotendinous ring), the wave of depolarization is delayed by approximately 0.1 s, so that the atria can contract fully.
4. Conduction continues through the bundle of His and its left and right bundle branches. These are very fast conduction pathways.
5. Numerous subendocardial Purkinje fibres distribute the impulse to the work cells in the endocardium.
6. Adjacent work cells then continue the spread to the epicardium to depolarize the whole ventricle.

All cells involved in the conduction process are muscle cells not nerves. They act as an electrical syncytium as they have low resistance electrical connections between them (gap junctions in the intercalated disc).

The SA node controls the heart rate because it has the fastest intrinsic firing rate, but the cells of the AV node and bundle of His can depolarize spontaneously at a slower rate if the SA node ceases to function. Sometimes this occurs in cases of heart block, where the impulse is not conducted properly through the fibrotendinous ring. Ventricular contraction then occurs at an independent rate (about 40 beats/min) to that of atrial contraction.

Fig. 2.36 Cardiac conduction pathway. The action potential is initiated in the sinoatrial (SA) node and spreads throughout both atria. It travels through the atrioventricular (AV) node, where it is delayed, and then to the bundle of His. From here it travels down the left and right bundle branches and into Purkinje fibres. The action potential is then spread throughout the ventricles.

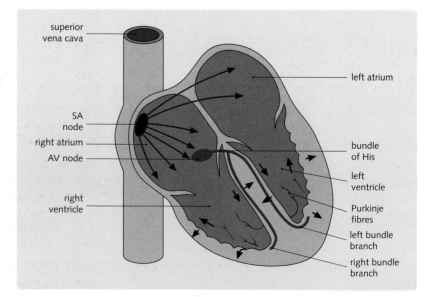

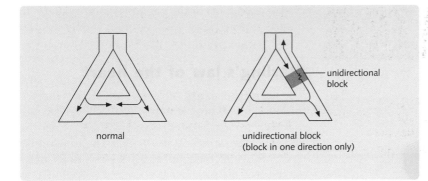

Fig. 2.37 Diagram illustrating heart block and re-entry. The direction of the impulse is indicated by the arrow. A block results from slow or absent conduction. Re-entry results from re-excitation of a region of the heart that has already contracted in the cardiac cycle. It depends upon the presence of a unidirectional block, and it is related to slow conduction and a short refractory period. (Redrawn with permission from Page C P et al (eds). Integrated pharmacology. London: Mosby, 1997.)

Heart block is said to occur if there is slow or absent conduction in an area of the myocardium. The action potential can take longer to reach an area of the myocardium and rhythm disturbances can, therefore, result. These are termed arrhythmias.

Re-entry occurs when the wave of depolarization travels back to re-excite an area of muscle that has already contracted (Fig. 2.37). This usually happens as a consequence of ischaemic damage to an area of myocardium. Again this may result in an arrhythmia (see Chapter 5).

Electrocardiography

The electrical activity of the heart can be measured by performing an electrocardiogram (ECG). This uses electrodes placed on the skin to detect the changing electrical potential within the tissue of the heart.

The characteristic elements of an ECG are:

- P wave – due to atrial depolarization.
- PR interval – from the onset of the P wave to the onset of the QRS complex (approximately 120–200 ms). This represents the time taken for atrial depolarization and the impulse to conduct through the AV node, His bundle and into the Purkinje fibres.
- QRS complex – due to ventricular depolarization (<120 ms).
- QT interval – the time taken from depolarization of the ventricles to the end of repolarization (approximately 400 ms).
- T wave – due to ventricular repolarization.

These can be related to the cardiac cycle (Fig. 2.34), and their significance is explained fully in Chapter 8.

Atrial fibrillation is a very common arrhythmia, usually brought about by ischaemic heart disease, valvular heart disease, alcohol or thyrotoxicosis. It causes the atria to fibrillate, hence losing the atrial component of cardiac filling. This results in a reduced efficiency of cardiac output, and a rapid ventricular rhythm to compensate. Treatment is centred on restoring sinus rhythm if possible, slowing the ventricular rate and prophylactic anticoagulation.

CONTROL OF CARDIAC OUTPUT

Definitions and concepts

Definitions include:

- Cardiac output (CO) – the volume of blood ejected by one ventricle in one minute.
- Stroke volume (SV) – the volume of blood ejected in one ventricular contraction.
- Stroke work (SW) – the amount of external energy expended in one ventricular contraction. SW is the mean arterial pressure (MAP) multiplied by the SV.

Total mechanical work equals the area within the pressure–volume loop. To calculate total energy expended, you must add internal work (i.e. work during isovolumetric contraction), external work (i.e. SW), and heat.

Other definitions are:

- Contractility – the force of contraction for a given fibre length.

- Heart rate (HR) – the number of ventricular contractions in one minute.
- End-diastolic volume (EDV) – the volume of blood in the ventricle just before contraction.
- End-diastolic pressure (EDP) – the pressure of blood in the ventricle just before contraction (preload – see below).
- End-systolic volume – the volume of blood left in the ventricle after contraction.
- Central venous pressure (CVP) – the pressure of blood in the great veins as they enter the right atrium.
- Venous return (VR) – the volume of blood returning to the right heart in one minute.
- Total peripheral resistance (TPR) – the resistance to the flow of blood in the whole system. It is MAP divided by the CO.
- Systemic vascular resistance (SVR) – the resistance to blood flow offered by all of the systemic vasculature, excluding the pulmonary vasculature. It is calculated as (MAP – Right Atrial Pressure) / CO.
- Ejection fraction – the proportion of EDV which is ejected by contraction.

The main equations governing CO and work are:

$$CO = SV \times HR$$
$$TPR = MAP / CO$$
$$SW = SV \times MAP$$
$$BP = CO \times SVR$$

Only two things directly affect CO:

- End-diastolic volume of the right heart (i.e. initial fibre length; this does not apply in pulmonary artery obstruction).
- Resistance to outflow.

As CO is a product of SV and HR, changes in SV will affect CO. SV is governed by:

- Initial stretch – see Starling's law (below).
- Contractility.
- MAP, which opposes ejection of blood.

The Fick principle states that the volume of oxygen taken up by the blood in the lungs, divided by the arteriovenous oxygen content difference, is equal to the cardiac output. This example utilizes the law of conservation of matter; what goes in must come out! Remember that cardiac output is therefore limited by venous return – without inte-

grated regulation of the cardiovascular system, an increased heart rate will be compensated by reduced stroke volume. This also applies in shock.

Starling's law of the heart

'The energy released during contraction depends upon the initial fibre length' (Fig. 2.38). The greater the heart is stretched by filling then the greater the energy released by contraction. This phenomenon is due to the stretch-dependent sensitivity of myocardial contractile proteins to Ca^{2+}, and it is known as Starling's law.

Although the initial stretch of the myocardium is produced by the EDV, EDP is easier to measure and the relationship between the two is almost linear. EDP plotted against SV produces the Starling curve (Fig. 2.39). Excessively high filling pressures will cause excessive distension and the relationship is no longer valid. EDP in the right ventricle is closely related to CVP.

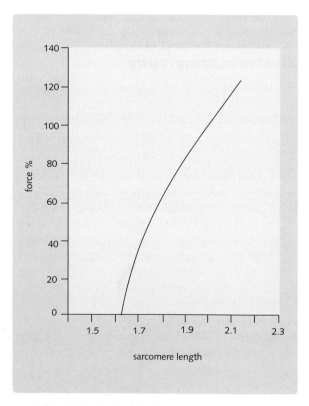

Fig. 2.38 Sarcomere length compared with tension. Increasing the initial sarcomere length increases tension, up to the maximum stretch possible for an individual myocyte.

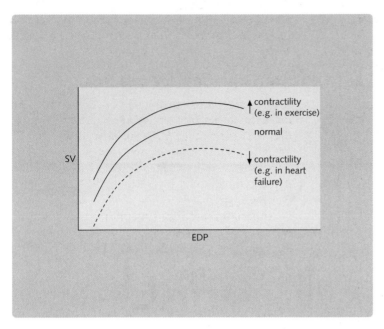

Fig. 2.39 Stroke volume (SV) compared with end-diastolic pressure (EDP). This produces the Starling curve, which shows that an increase in EDP (and therefore end-diastolic volume (EDV) as they have an almost linear relationship) causes an increased SV. There is, however, a limit at which the curve turns downwards and the relationship is no longer valid. The mechanism for this downturn is complex, and it mainly reflects excessive dilatation of the ventricle and valvular regurgitation. Changes in contractility are characterized by upward (positively inotropic) and downward (negatively inotropic) displacement of the Starling curve.

Starling's law matches right and left ventricular stroke volumes. If HR and myocardial contractility are constant, CVP will determine the CO. Although CVP affects the right ventricle, within a few beats the venous pressure will change in the pulmonary circulation and so the filling pressure of the left ventricle will also be affected, and left ventricular output will change according to the stretch produced by the new EDV. Remember that the circulatory system is closed, with the two ventricles in series. Cardiac output must equal venous return, and discrepancies between left and right ventricular output can only be transient in the steady state. Pathological changes may produce inequalities, such as left-sided (or congestive) heart failure producing pulmonary oedema.

Preload and afterload are important factors affecting stroke volume, and hence CO. Although the ideas originate from isolated muscle experiments, they have been applied to the study of the heart in vivo:

- Preload is the force associated with the degree of initial stretch in the ventricle from the initial volume load. It is determined by the EDV, which is related to EDP. In the right side of the heart, EDP is almost equal to CVP.

- Afterload is the force (load in systole) that is determined by MAP (which is related to the resistance to outflow, i.e. TPR) and ventricular volume by the Laplace relationship.

An increase in preload will increase CO according to Starling's law. An increase in afterload will initially decrease CO. The heart will have a greater residual volume after contraction. If the filling pressure remains constant, the greater residual volume will distend the ventricle further and the next contraction will be stronger. This is an attempt to restore the CO.

Starling's experiments were conducted on an isolated heart–lung preparation in 1914 (Fig. 2.40). While it is not possible to monitor the determinants of CO in the way Starling could by isolating the heart and lungs, cardiologists can insert a single catheter from the femoral artery back up the aorta and into the left ventricle by passing it retrograde through the aortic valve. The catheter contains conductance sensors to measure left ventricular volume and a pressure sensor at the tip. This freely records the pressure–volume loops (Fig. 2.41).

Starling's findings in the controlled situation of the isolated heart–lung preparation are important

Fig. 2.40 Starling heart–lung preparation. He used an isolated heart–lung preparation and looked at the result of varying end-diastolic volume (EDV) and arterial resistance. EDV is sometimes called preload; arterial resistance is sometimes termed afterload. These terms were not used by Starling in his experiments, but they are frequently used now. (Redrawn with permission of the Physiological Society.)

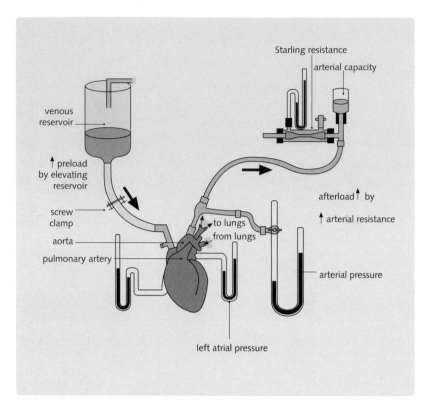

in enabling clinicians to understand the importance of:

- Adequate, but not excessive, filling of the ventricles (e.g. in heart failure, high EDV may be pathological).
- Keeping peripheral resistance as low as possible to maximize CO.
- Maintaining a sufficient level of contractility to maintain life when the previous determinants have been optimized.

When the blood supply through the coronary arteries is compromised it is important to keep certain methods of increasing CO (especially increased contractility) to a minimum, because they increase oxygen consumption of the heart muscle, and therefore increase the demand for blood supply and the intensity of ischaemia.

Factors affecting contractility

A change in contractility can take place as a result of the action of various factors affecting the myocyte (Fig. 2.42). The energy of contraction is affected by other variables in addition to that of initial fibre length (Starling mechanism; Fig. 2.39). The term inotropic is also used to denote the contractility of the heart. Positive inotropes (increased contractility) include:

- Sympathetic stimulation. Adrenaline and noradrenaline from sympathetic nerves bind to β_1-receptors on myocytes and increase intracellular Ca^{2+} by cyclic adenosine monophosphate (cAMP)-activated protein kinase A and G-protein linked Ca^{2+} channels. This increases the force of contraction and shortens systole.
- Plasma Ca^{2+}. Increases in plasma Ca^{2+} result in increased sarcoplasmic Ca^{2+} in the myocytes.
- pH.
- Increased temperature.
- Drugs: cardiac glycosides – digoxin, ouabain; β-agonists – adrenaline, isoprenaline; and most antiarrhythmics.

Negative inotropes include:

- Disease (e.g. ischaemia, hypoxia).
- Acidity.
- Drugs: β-blockers (e.g. propranolol), Ca^{2+}-channel blockers (e.g. verapamil), barbiturates, and most anaesthetic agents.

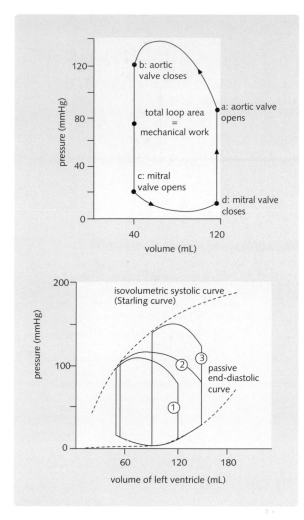

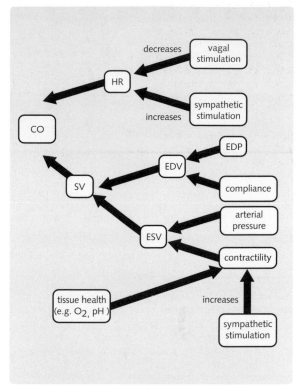

Fig. 2.42 Summary of the factors affecting cardiac output (CO, cardiac output; EDP, end-diastolic pressure; EDV, end-diastolic volume; HR, heart rate; ESV, end-systolic volume; SV, stroke volume).

Fig. 2.41 Pressure–volume loops (1, normal state; 2, increased end-diastolic volume (EDV) leads to increased stroke volume (SV) if arterial pressure is constant; 3, Increased EDV and Increased MAP result In a decreased SV). The end-systolic points of the loops produce the Starling curve so long as the contractility remains constant.

Venous return, central venous pressure, and cardiac output

Venous return (VR) depends on the mean circulatory pressure (P_{mc}), right atrial pressure (P_{ra}) and venous resistance (R_v) according to the following formula:

$$VR = (P_{mc} - P_{ra}) / R_v$$

Right atrial pressure is equivalent to the central venous pressure. The mean circulatory pressure is experimentally derived, and is the pressure that

would result throughout the circulatory system if the heart were to stop beating. It is determined principally by the blood volume and the degree of sympathetic activation (Fig. 2.43). The effect of sympathetic activation is to increase the 'tightness' with which blood is constrained within the circulatory system, but this should not be confused with TPR, as this is a separate and distinct variable.

The equation is the equivalent of the previous description of arterial blood flow, i.e. flow (venous return) is equal to the pressure gradient between the central veins and the systemic circulation divided by the resistance. In health, any changes are automatically compensated. For example, an increased right atrial pressure leads to reduced venous return, but it also leads to an increased output by Starling's law. This will then reduce the right atrial pressure, restoring equilibrium. There may be a transient discrepancy between venous

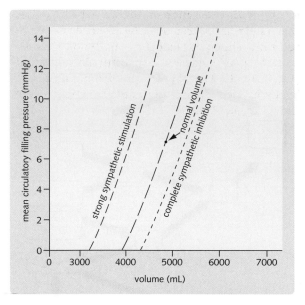

Fig. 2.43 The effects of volume and sympathetic activation on the mean circulatory filling pressure (P_{mc}). The mean filling pressure depends on the degree of filling (volume) and the stiffness of the compartment, often referred to as the tone. The reciprocal of the stiffness is called capacitance, compliance, or distensibility. The tone is increased by sympathetic stimulation, which shifts the curve to the left (vasoconstriction/venoconstriction) so that there is a higher filling pressure for a given volume. (Redrawn with permission from Guyton A C, Hall J E. Textbook of medical physiology, 9th edn. London: W B Saunders, 1995.)

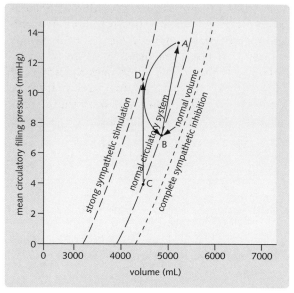

Fig. 2.44 Examples of compensatory changes in mean circulatory filling pressure in disease. Compensatory changes in chronic heart disease (A), where volume increases and sympathetic stimulation increases mean filling pressure. Treatment is to counter these changes and unload the heart (B). In haemorrhagic shock (C), the blood loss is countered by sympathetic activation (D) (see Fig. 2.45).

return and cardiac output (as strictly defined), but remember that compensation occurs automatically. If the right atrial pressure remains raised, increased sympathetic activity will increase the mean filling pressure to compensate, producing a new equilibrium with a higher CVP and a higher cardiac output.

Following haemorrhage the cardiovascular system undergoes many changes to maintain adequate pressure to perfuse the vital organs, including vasoconstriction, an increase in heart rate and venous return. Starling's law helps us understand the body's physiological response to injury, and also the direct effects of treatments we provide, such as fluid (increasing preload), and inotropes.

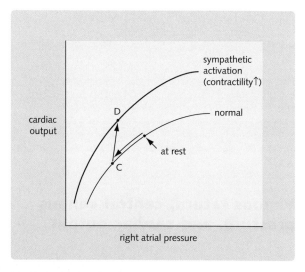

Fig. 2.45 Cardiac function curve showing the changes in haemorrhagic shock. Fluid loss causes a fall in cardiac filling (C), reducing right atrial pressure. Cardiac output will then fall, but increased sympathetic activity will increase contractility (moving the Starling curve upward and to the left) while also causing venoconstriction which will increase venous return and hence raise right atrial pressure.

The effects of disease and resulting compensatory changes are shown in Fig. 2.44. In right-sided heart disease, where myocardial function is compromised and right atrial pressure is persistently raised, the body compensates by increasing sympathetic drive and retaining fluid to increase blood volume (Fig. 2.44, A). A common treatment for this situation is nitrate, which relaxes the system as indicated in Fig. 2.44, B. In hypovolaemic shock, a reduction in blood volume is also associated with sympathetic activation (Fig. 2.44, C, D). The effects of the changes in hypovolaemic shock on cardiac function are shown in Fig. 2.45.

Structure and function of the vessels

Objectives

You should be able to:

- Describe the functional and anatomical classifications of vessels.
- Describe the anatomy and histology of a typical vessel.
- Describe the main arterial supply and venous drainage to the body.
- Understand the embryology and development of the fetal circulation.
- Explain the basis for the changes in vascular resistance through the vascular tree, and how these changes affect blood pressure and the velocity of blood flow.
- Measure blood pressure manually and interpret Korotkoff sounds.
- Recall the intrinsic factors which affect blood pressure.
- Define the laws of Poiseuille, Ohm and Laplace.
- Understand the forces acting on a capillary bed.
- Understand what affects venous and lymphatic flow.

ORGANIZATION OF THE VESSELS

Classification of the vessels

The circulatory system is composed of vessels designed for:

- Conductance.
- Resistance.
- Exchange.
- Capacitance.

Conductance

These are low-resistance vessels, which are arteries with predominantly elastic walls. Their role is delivery of blood to more distal vessels, although they also have a small resistance role.

Resistance

These vessels are the terminal arteries and arterioles, and they are the main resistance to blood flow.

Resistance vessels act to control local blood flow. Dilatation of these vessels lowers resistance and increases blood flow (vasodilatation). Constriction of these vessels increases resistance and decreases blood flow (vasoconstriction). They can, therefore, influence the exchange vessels by governing the flow that reaches them.

Exchange

These vessels are the numerous capillaries that have very thin walls. This optimizes their function, which is to allow rapid transfer between blood and tissues. They also contribute some resistance to flow.

Capacitance

These vessels are thin-walled, low-resistance venules and veins. They act as a variable reservoir of blood and contain almost two-thirds of the blood volume. These veins are innervated by venoconstrictor fibres which, when stimulated, can displace the blood back towards the heart.

> The components of a vessel wall reflect that vessel's function. For example, if an arterial wall contains many more elastic fibres than collagen fibres, it will be more compliant than other vessels and better suited to act as a conductance vessel.

35

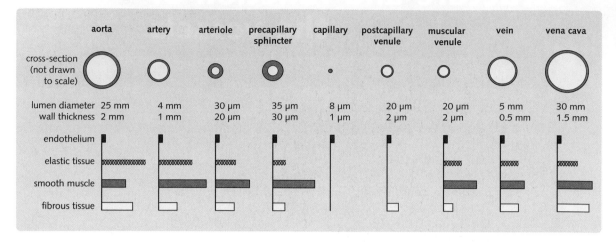

Fig. 3.1 Vessels of the circulation (Adapted with permission from Burton A C, Physiol Rev. 34: 619, 1954).

Vasculature

The vasculature (Fig. 3.1) is classified anatomically into:

- Elastic arteries (e.g. aorta and common carotids).
- Muscular arteries (e.g. coronary, cerebral, and popliteal arteries).
- Arterioles.
- Capillaries.
- Postcapillary venules.
- Muscular venules.
- Veins.

The main function of the arteries and arterioles is to deliver blood to the capillaries. In the capillaries, exchange with and filtration into the interstitial fluid takes place. Fluid and metabolites return to the heart through veins and lymphatic vessels. Veins return blood to the heart and the lymphatic system returns excess filtrate (lymph) to the blood.

Anatomy of the circulatory system

The anatomy of the circulatory system is shown in Figs 3.2–3.14.

Cerebrovascular disease is the most common neurological problem experienced in the western world. It occurs as the result of clot deposition, or more rarely from a bleed, in the Circle of Willis. The circle, being a complete anastomosis, allows blood to flow irrespective of a small blockage, minimizing the neurological insult of the stroke.

The artery of Adamkiewicz is important as it supplies the anterior spinal cord. If this becomes damaged, for example from a dissection (tear) of the aorta, it can result in paralysis.

Development of the circulation

The vasculature develops from the angioblastic cords of mesoderm. The aortic ends of the primitive heart tube become the aortic arches and dorsal aortae. The aortic arches develop into the great arteries of the neck and thorax, whereas the dorsal aortae produce the following branches:

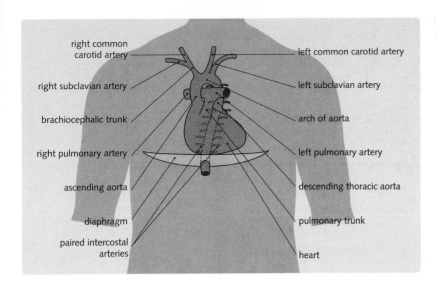

Fig. 3.2 Arterial supply of the thorax.

right common carotid artery

right subclavian artery

brachiocephalic trunk

right pulmonary artery

ascending aorta

diaphragm

paired intercostal arteries

left common carotid artery

left subclavian artery

arch of aorta

left pulmonary artery

descending thoracic aorta

pulmonary trunk

heart

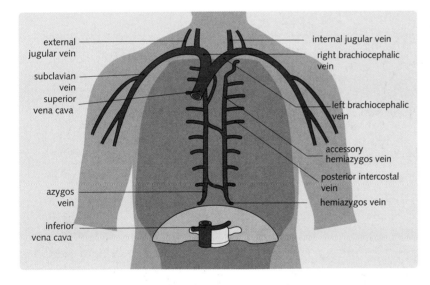

Fig. 3.3 Venous drainage of the thorax.

external jugular vein

subclavian vein

superior vena cava

azygos vein

inferior vena cava

internal jugular vein

right brachiocephalic vein

left brachiocephalic vein

accessory hemiazygos vein

posterior intercostal vein

hemiazygos vein

- Ventral branches (derived from the remnants of the vitelline arteries), which supply the gastrointestinal tract.
- Lateral branches, which supply retroperitoneal structures (e.g. kidneys).
- Intersegmental branches, which supply the rest of the body.

The paired dorsal aortae connect to the umbilical arteries, which carry blood to the placenta. The venous system consists of three components, which are initially paired:

- Cardinal system, which drains the head, neck, body wall, and limbs.
- Vitelline veins, which drain the yolk sac.
- Umbilical veins, which carry blood from the placenta to the embryo.

Initially, the venous system drains into the sinus horns, and subsequently into the venae cavae and right atrium. In general, it is the right-sided veins that persist while the left-sided veins regress during gestation, and so systemic venous drainage is via the vena cava to the right side of the heart.

Fig. 3.4 Arterial supply of the abdomen.

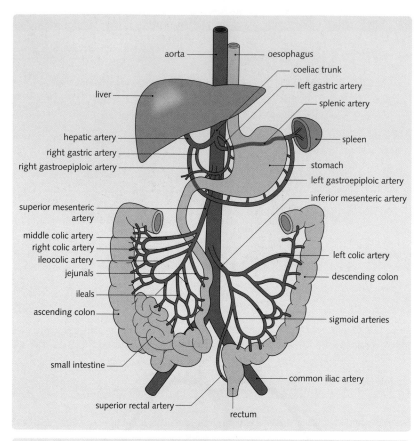

Fig. 3.5 Venous drainage of the abdomen.

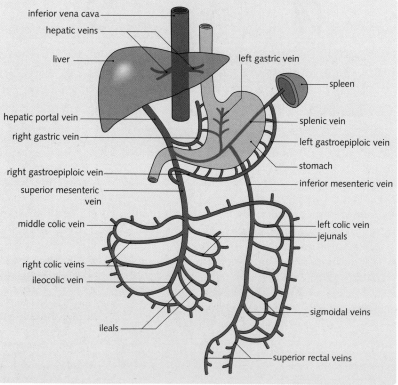

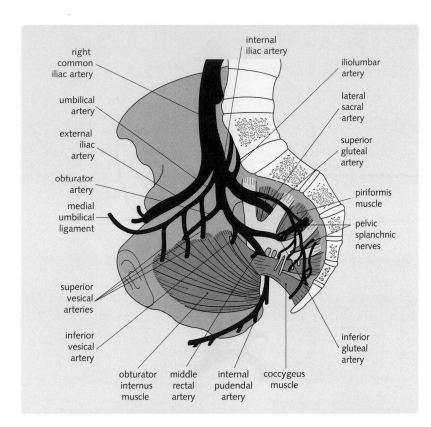

Fig. 3.6 Vessels of the pelvis.

internal
iliac artery

right
common
iliac artery

umbilical
artery

external
iliac
artery

obturator
artery

medial
umbilical
ligament

superior
vesical
arteries

inferior
vesical
artery

obturator
internus
muscle

middle
rectal
artery

internal
pudendal
artery

coccygeus
muscle

iliolumbar
artery

lateral
sacral
artery

superior
gluteal
artery

piriformis
muscle

pelvic
splanchnic
nerves

inferior
gluteal
artery

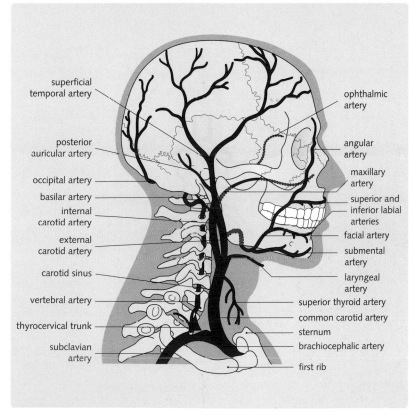

Fig. 3.7 Arteries of the neck and head.

superficial
temporal artery

posterior
auricular artery

occipital artery

basilar artery

internal
carotid artery

external
carotid artery

carotid sinus

vertebral artery

thyrocervical trunk

subclavian
artery

ophthalmic
artery

angular
artery

maxillary
artery

superior and
inferior labial
arteries

facial artery

submental
artery

laryngeal
artery

superior thyroid artery

common carotid artery

sternum

brachiocephalic artery

first rib

Fig. 3.8 Veins of the neck and head.

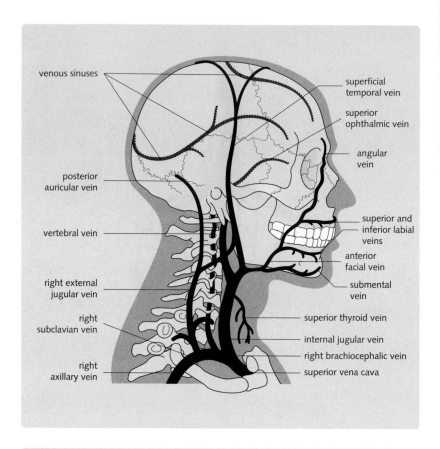

Fig. 3.9 Arteries of the brain. The Circle of Willis is an anastomotic loop constructed from the anterior and posterior communicating, and anterior and posterior cerebral arteries. The cranial nerves are also shown.

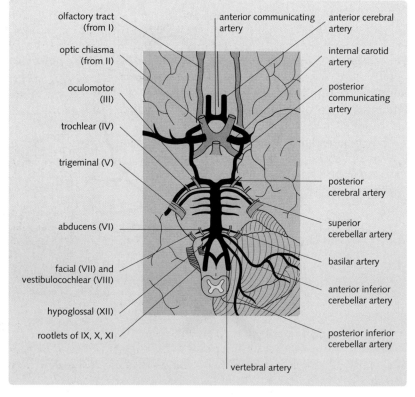

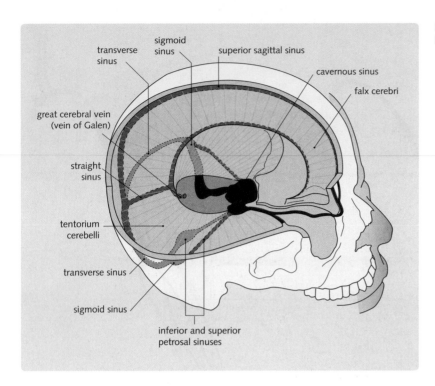

Fig. 3.10 Venous drainage of the brain.

Labels on figure:
- transverse sinus
- sigmoid sinus
- superior sagittal sinus
- cavernous sinus
- falx cerebri
- great cerebral vein (vein of Galen)
- straight sinus
- tentorium cerebelli
- transverse sinus
- sigmoid sinus
- inferior and superior petrosal sinuses

However, it is the left umbilical vein that persists while the right umbilical vein disappears.

Within the liver, the vitelline system forms the ductus venosus, shunting blood from the umbilical vein directly into the inferior vena cava during gestation. This is vital, as it allows oxygenated blood to enter the right atrium of the heart, pass predominantly through the foramen ovale and then be pumped around the fetus (Fig. 3.15).

The foramen ovale enables the oxygenated blood in the right atrium to pass into the left atrium and reach the systemic circulation, bypassing the pulmonary circulation.

The ductus arteriosus develops from the sixth aortic arch. It connects the pulmonary arteries to the descending aorta. This allows oxygenated blood pumped into the pulmonary arteries (i.e. blood not shunted through the foramen ovale) to enter the systemic circulation. This is necessary as the lungs are not functional during gestation, negating the need for a large pulmonary circulation. The duct is kept open during fetal life by circulating prostaglandins, and this stimulation may be continued artificially early in the neonatal period.

The head receives a preferential blood supply, so if there is a decrease in umbilical artery supply the head will continue to receive an adequate blood supply at the expense of the rest of the body (i.e. the head grows but the body does not).

Deoxygenated blood returns to the placenta through the umbilical arteries, which connect to the aorta.

Multiple measurements are taken at ultrasound scan in pregnant women, including Doppler flow studies of the umbilical vessels, and head/abdomen circumference ratio. If there is decreased arterial supply, intra-uterine growth retardation (IUGR) can be predicted and monitored by serial measurements showing a failure in growth of abdominal circumference.

Circulatory adaptations at birth

A series of changes convert the single system of blood flow around the fetus into dual systems at birth.

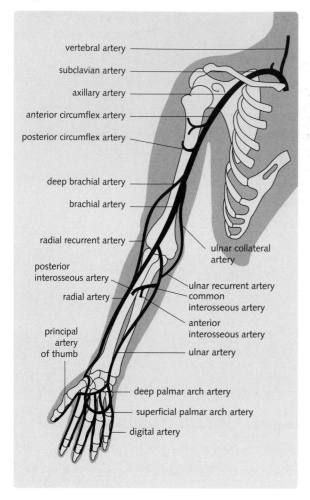

Fig. 3.11 Arterial supply of the upper limbs.

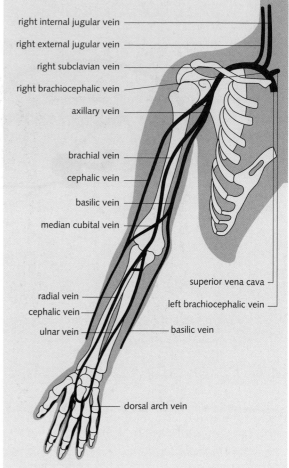

Fig. 3.12 Venous drainage of the upper limbs.

Blood flow in the umbilical vessels drastically declines in the first few minutes after birth because of:

• Compression of the cord.
• Vasoconstriction in response to cold, mechanical stimuli, and circulating fetal catecholamines as a result of the stress of descending through the birth canal.

At birth, the pulmonary vascular resistance falls rapidly because:

• The thorax of the fetus is compressed on descent, emptying the amniotic fluid from the lungs.
• The mechanical effect of ventilation opens the constricted alveolar vessels.

• Raising P_{O_2} and lowering P_{CO_2} causes vasodilatation of the pulmonary vessels.

This produces an increase in the pulmonary blood flow.

The sudden cessation of umbilical blood flow and the opening of the pulmonary system causes a change in the pressure balance in the atria. There is a pressure drop in the right atrium and a pressure rise in the left atrium (caused by an increased pulmonary venous return to the left atrium). This changes the pressure gradient across the atria and forces the flexible septum primum against the rigid septum secundum, closing the foramen ovale. These two septa fuse together after about 3 months.

Fig. 3.13 Arterial supply of the lower limbs.

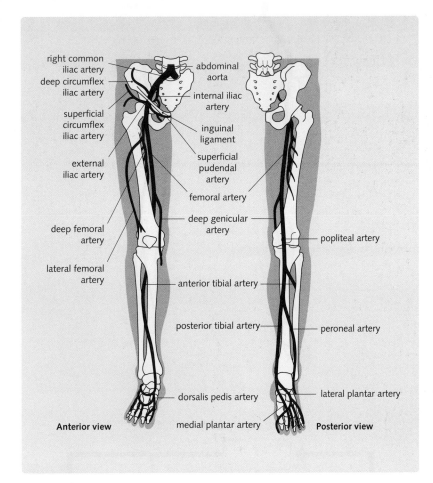

right common
iliac artery

deep circumflex
iliac artery

superficial
circumflex
iliac artery

external
iliac artery

deep femoral
artery

lateral femoral
artery

abdominal
aorta

internal iliac
artery

inguinal
ligament

superficial
pudendal
artery

femoral artery

deep genicular
artery

popliteal artery

anterior tibial artery

posterior tibial artery

peroneal artery

dorsalis pedis artery

lateral plantar artery

Anterior view

medial plantar artery

Posterior view

The ductus venosus closes soon after birth (Figs 3.16 and 3.17). The mechanism is unclear, but it is thought to involve prostaglandin inhibition. The closure is not vital to life, as the umbilical vein no longer carries any blood.

The ductus arteriosus closes 1–8 days after birth. It is thought that as the pulmonary circulation fills, the pressure drop in the pulmonary trunk causes blood to flow from the aorta into the pulmonary trunk through the ductus arteriosus. This blood is oxygenated and the increase in PO_2 causes the smooth muscle in the wall of the ductus to constrict, obstructing the flow in the ductus arteriosus. Eventually, the intima of the ductus arteriosus thickens – complete obliteration of the ductus results in the formation of the ligamentum arteriosum, which attaches the pulmonary trunk to the aorta.

Congenital vascular abnormalities

Many circulatory anomalies can develop, but few of these conditions cause any problems. Those that do include:

- Patent ductus arteriosus – failure of the duct to close in the neonatal period.
- Coarctation of the aorta – an abnormal stenotic thickening of the aorta that affects systemic blood flow and causes upper body hypertension.
- Persistent patent foramen ovale – a very common failure of fusion of the septum primum and secundum, which in the presence of a raised right atrial pressure may lead to a permanent atrial shunt.

Fig. 3.14 Venous drainage of the lower limbs.

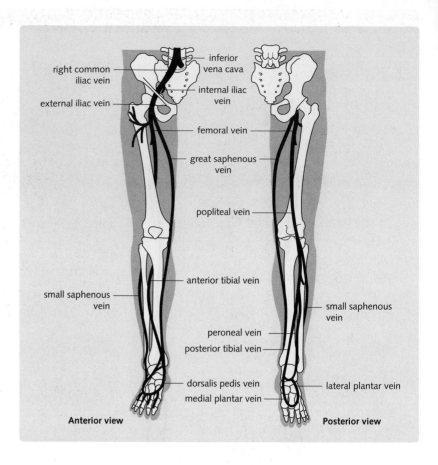

Fig. 3.15 Fetal blood pathway.

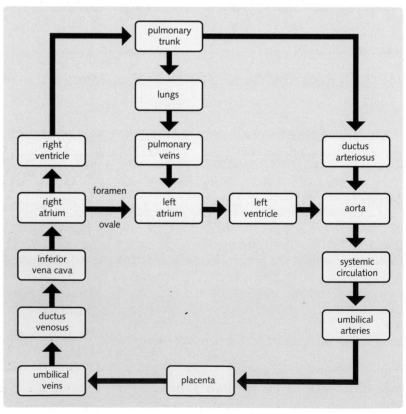

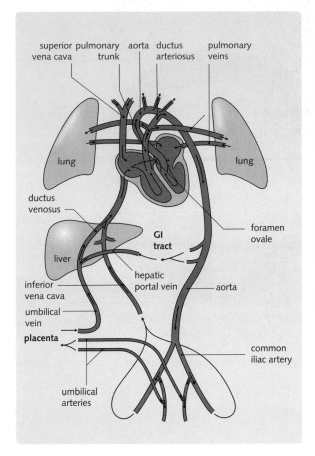

Fig. 3.16 Fetal circulation in utero.

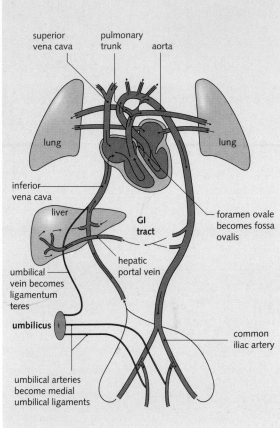

Fig. 3.17 Neonatal circulation shortly after birth. Note the closure of the foramen ovale, ductus arteriosus, ductus venosus, and umbilical vessels closing off the fetal shunts.

There are many other congenital cardiac defects, further information on which may be found in Chapter 5.

Structure and histology

A blood vessel has an endothelium surrounded by three main layers (or tunicae). These are termed the intima, media, and adventitia. Fig. 3.18 shows the layers of a typical vessel.

Arteries and veins

An elastic artery consists of concentric layers of elastic and smooth muscle, whereas a muscular artery has prominent muscular media, with internal and external elastic laminae. In contrast, veins have a very thin media. Fig. 3.19 shows the structure of an elastic artery, a muscular artery, and a vein.

There are a number of small vessels (vasa nervorum) which supply nerves in the body. In certain conditions, such as diabetes, these vessels are targeted. As such, the nerves become damaged and a neuropathy develops. The neuropathy then predisposes to subsequent joint damage and ulceration.

Capillary

The structure of a capillary is shown in Fig. 3.20.

Lymphatic vessel

The structure of a lymphatic capillary is shown in Fig. 3.21.

Fig. 3.18 Cross-section of a generic vessel showing the distinction between layers.

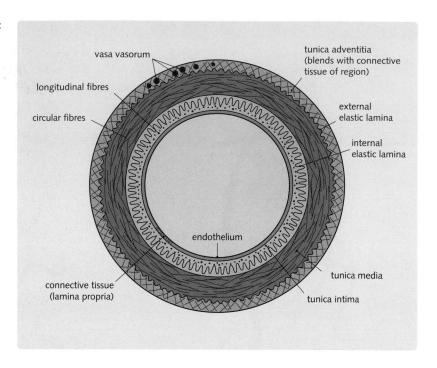

Fig. 3.19 Cross-sections through walls of elastic arteries, muscular arteries, and veins.

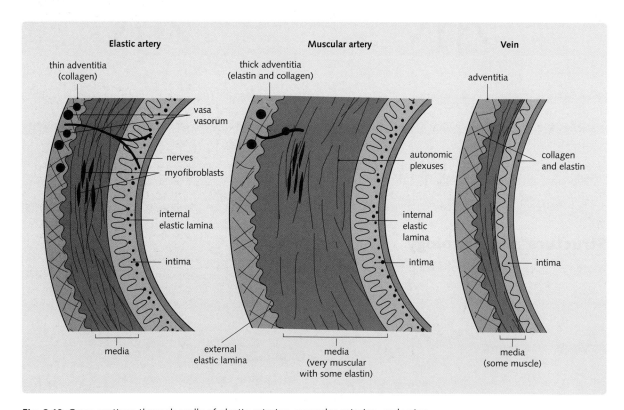

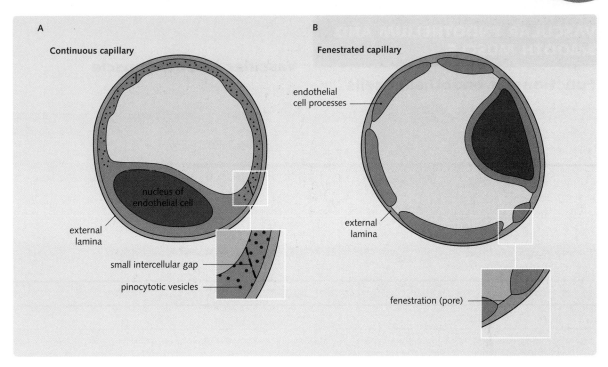

Fig. 3.20 Cross-sections of capillaries with continuous and fenestrated walls. Continuous capillary walls are less permeable than fenestrated capillary walls. (Redrawn with permission from Stevens A, Lowe J. Human histology. London: Mosby, 1997.)

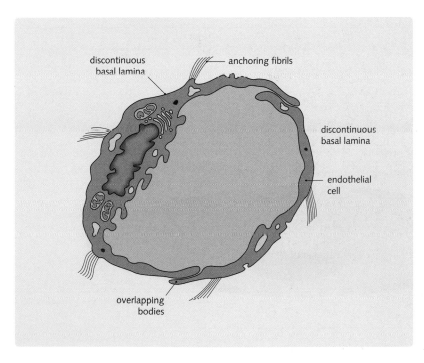

Fig. 3.21 Cross-section of a lymph capillary. Lymph capillaries only allow flow into the lumen but not out. Overlapping endothelial cells operate as one-way valves to accomplish this. The anchoring filaments connect the endothelial cells to the surrounding tissue. When surrounding tissues are swollen with excess interstitial fluid (e.g. in inflammation) the filaments pull the endothelial cells apart to increase lymphatic flow. The discontinuous basal lamina (basement membrane) also allows greater movement of fluids and solutes.

VASCULAR ENDOTHELIUM AND SMOOTH MUSCLE

Functions of endothelial cells

Endothelial cells (see Fig. 3.35) are involved in:

- Transportation of substances between interstitium and plasma.
- Providing a friction-free surface.
- Regulation of haemostasis and fibrinolysis.
- Inflammatory responses.
- Control of vascular tone.

Some of these functions require the secretion of a variety of substances (Fig. 3.22).

Vascular smooth muscle

Structure

The structure of smooth muscle is shown in Fig. 3.23. A mass of smooth muscle functions as if it were a single unit.

Contraction of vascular smooth muscle

Contraction is initiated by a rise in intracellular Ca^{2+}. This leads to an actin–myosin interaction,

Secreted factors and their functions	
Factor secreted	**Function**
Structural components	To form the basal lamina
Prostacyclin	Vasodilatation; inhibits platelet aggregation
Nitric oxide	Vasodilatation; inhibits platelet adhesion and aggregation
Angiotensin converting enzyme	Converts angiotensin I to II; degrades bradykinin and serotonin
Platelet activating factor	Activates platelets and neutrophils
Tissue plasminogen activator (tPA)	Regulates fibrinolysis
Thromboplastin	Promotes coagulation
Von Willebrand's factor	Promotes platelet adhesion and clotting

Fig. 3.22 Secreted factors from endothelial cells and their functions.

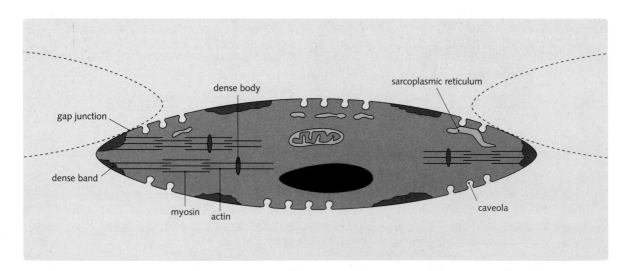

Fig. 3.23 Structure of a smooth muscle cell. The actin–myosin filaments have been magnified. (Adapted from Levick R. Introducing cardiovascular physiology. Butterworth-Heinemann, 1995. Reproduced by permission of Edward Arnold Ltd.)

which causes shortening and tension. The process differs from that in the myocardium in the following ways:

- Myosin light chain phosphorylation. Unlike skeletal or cardiac muscle, the myosin in vascular smooth muscle only becomes active if its light chains are phosphorylated. The enzyme is activated by a calcium–calmodulin complex, which is dependent on a rise in intracellular Ca^{2+} for its formation.
- Sustained actin–myosin interactions enable vascular smooth muscle to maintain tension for 0.3% of the energy needed by skeletal muscle. The actin–myosin interactions are long-lasting because of slow myosin kinetics.
- Sensitivity to intracellular Ca^{2+}. Chemical factors can alter the relationship between

cytoplasmic Ca^{2+} and contractile force (i.e. the sensitivity of the contractile apparatus to Ca^{2+} can be changed). The cytoplasmic Ca^{2+} concentration and the resting membrane potential are dependent upon the state of ion-conducting channels (K^+, Ca^{2+}, and Cl^- channels).

Effect of sympathetic innervation

Fig. 3.24 shows the mechanism of sympathetic innervation.

Vascular smooth muscle relaxation

Vascular smooth muscle relaxation can be brought about by four different mechanisms. Each mechanism relies upon reducing intracellular Ca^{2+}:

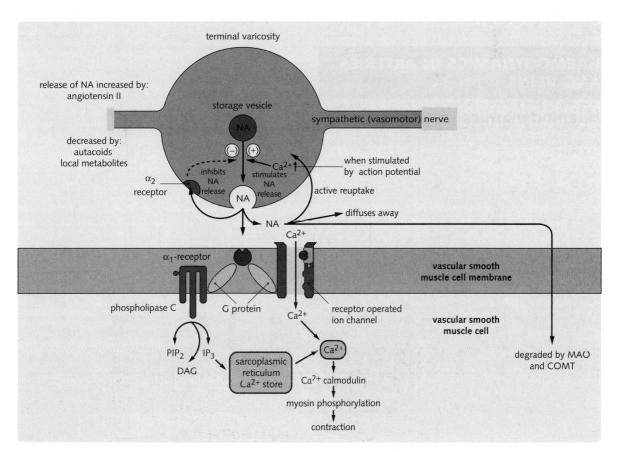

Fig. 3.24 Release of noradrenaline (NA) from a sympathetic junction and its effect on the vascular smooth muscle (VSM) cell. Sympathetic stimulation results in the release of NA from the sympathetic terminal varicosities. NA acts on (amongst others) α_1-receptors on the VSM cells. This results in an increase in intracellular Ca^{2+} by directly opening Ca^{2+} channels and via a second messenger system releasing Ca^{2+} from the sarcoplasmic reticulum. It is the increase of intracellular Ca^{2+} that brings about contraction (AP, action potential; COMT, catechol O-methyltransferase; DAG, diacylglycerol; IP_3, inositol triphosphate; MAO, monoamine oxidase; PIP_2, phosphatidyl inositol bisphosphate).

- Hyperpolarization. Hyperpolarizing the resting membrane reduces the number of open Ca^{2+} channels, leading to a decrease in intracellular Ca^{2+} concentration and relaxation. Hyperpolarization is caused by hypoxia, acidosis, drugs (e.g. diazoxide, cromakalim, pinacidil) and numerous peptides, including endothelium-derived hyperpolarizing factor, calcitotin-gene-related peptide, substance P and bradykinin acetylcholine.
- Cyclic adenosine monophosphate (cAMP)-mediated vasodilatation (Fig. 3.25).
- Cyclic guanosine monophosphate (cGMP)-mediated vasodilatation (Fig. 3.26).
- Altered sensitivity to intracellular Ca^{2+}. A lowered sensitivity of the contractile apparatus to the cytoplasmic Ca^{2+} makes the contraction weaker for a given concentration of Ca^{2+} and causes dilatation.

HAEMODYNAMICS IN ARTERIES AND VEINS

Haemodynamics in arteries

In normal arteries and veins, there is laminar flow (Fig. 3.27). Turbulent flow occurs in the ventricles.

'Single-file' flow occurs in capillaries. Although this is a simplistic view it is sufficient for most basic purposes.

Pulse waveform

The difference between systolic and diastolic pressure is termed the pulse pressure. The pressure wave created by ventricular ejection depends upon:

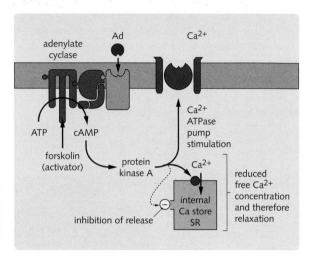

Fig. 3.25 cAMP-mediated vasodilatation as shown by the action of adrenaline (Ad) (ATP, adenosine triphosphate; SR, sarcoplasmic reticulum).

Fig. 3.26 cGMP-mediated vasodilatation as shown by the action of vasoactive mediators (ADP, adenosine diphosphate; GTP, guanosine triphosphate; NO, nitric oxide; VSM cell, vascular smooth muscle cell).

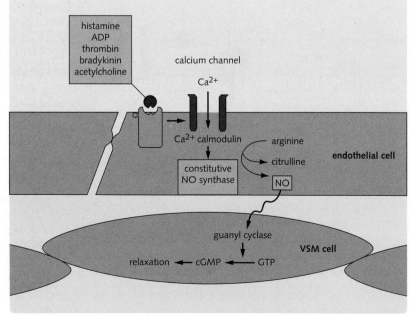

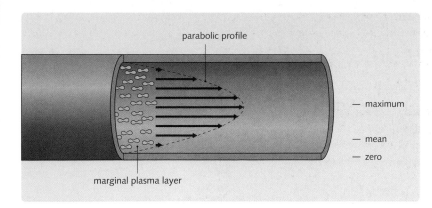

Fig. 3.27 The dynamics of laminar flow. Blood flows as if in sheets (laminae) with blood being faster in the middle than at the sides, where friction slows flow. The dashed line indicates the parabolic profile of the different speeds across the vessel. Cells tend to accumulate in the centre of the flow, leaving a marginal plasma layer with fewer red cells at the periphery.

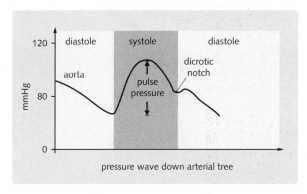

Fig. 3.28 Pulse waveform. The dicrotic notch is caused by closure of the aortic valve.

- Stroke volume.
- Heart rate.
- Compliance of the arterial wall.
- Peripheral resistance (afterload).
- Blood volume returning to the heart (preload).

The mean arterial pressure (MAP) is the arterial pressure averaged over time. The MAP is not just midway between diastolic and systolic pressure, as more time is spent in diastole than in systole (Fig. 3.28). Thus, MAP is closer to diastolic pressure, and is commonly approximated as one third of the pulse pressure added to diastolic pressure. The MAP is an important measurement to consider as it reflects organ perfusion more accurately than either systolic or diastolic blood pressure measurements.

Measurement of arterial blood pressure

Arterial blood pressure can be measured directly by using invasive catheters. However, it is usual prac-tice in most patients to measure blood pressure indi-rectly using a sphygmomanometer.

The sphygmomanometer is used as follows:

1. A suitably sized cuff is wrapped around the upper arm of the patient, who should be sitting or lying with the sphygmomanometer at the level of their heart.
2. The radial or brachial pulse is palpated, and the cuff inflated until the pulse is no longer palpable. This is an estimation of the systolic blood pressure.
3. The brachial artery is auscultated at the medial side of the antecubital fossa with a stethoscope. No sound should be heard.
4. The cuff pressure is gradually lowered (1–2 mmgHg/second) until a dull tapping sound is heard. The measurement taken at this time is the systolic pressure.
5. Further lowering of the cuff pressure results in louder sounds until the sounds suddenly become quieter, and then disappear. The measurement taken at this time is the diastolic pressure.

There are a number of audible stages when man-ually measuring blood pressure, known as the Korotkoff sounds:

I. Sharp thud (taken to be systolic blood pressure).
II. Loud blowing sound.
III. Soft thud.
IV. Soft blowing sound (occasionally used as diastolic blood pressure, e.g. in pregnancy).
V. Onset of silence (taken to be diastolic blood pressure).

Normal blood pressure

Normal blood pressure for a healthy adult male at rest is 120/80 mmHg. However, this value can vary with many factors, all of which must be taken into account when assessing a patient's blood pressure:

- Ageing causes an increase in blood pressure because of decreased arterial compliance secondary to arteriosclerosis. As a rough rule, systolic pressure should be equal to 100 mmHg plus age in years.
- During sleep, blood pressure falls because of the body's decreased metabolic demands.
- Heavy dynamic exercise increases blood pressure because of increased cardiac output. However, the increase in blood pressure is less than 30% because of decreased total peripheral resistance.
- Heavy static exercise greatly increases blood pressure (possibly, by more than 30%) because of the exercise pressor response.
- Anger, sexual excitement, and stress increase blood pressure, all because of sympathetically mediated responses.

Other factors that may cause changes in blood pressure include:

- Respiration. In the young, mean arterial pressure falls by a small amount during inspiration because of a transient fall in stroke volume.
- Pregnancy. Blood pressure falls gradually in the first trimester, reaching a minimum in the second trimester, and then rises to normal in the third trimester.
- Physiological processes. For example, the Valsalva manoeuvre and the diving reflex.
- Pathological processes. For example, shock, haemorrhage, and heart failure.

There is a physiological fall in blood pressure from the major arteries through the vascular tree. Note that the largest pressure drop is at arteriolar level, the site of the main resistance to blood flow (Fig. 3.29).

Blood flow and velocity

Blood flow is defined as the volume of blood that flows through a given tissue in a given time. For the whole body, this must equal the cardiac output. Ohm's law states:

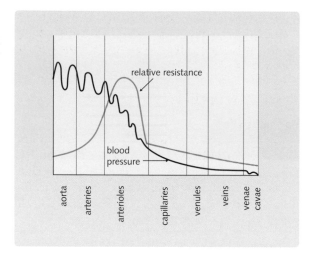

Fig. 3.29 How blood pressure and vascular resistance change across the vascular system. Pressure in the arterial side and in the great veins varies with the cardiac cycle.

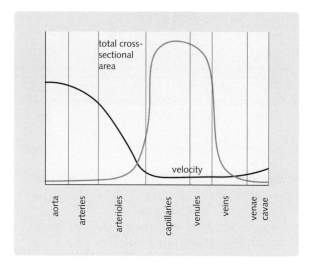

Fig. 3.30 Total cross-sectional area and mean velocity within the different anatomical classifications of vessels. Velocity in the arterial side actually varies with the cardiac cycle – the mean cycle is shown.

Flow = (Pressure difference) / resistance (I = V/R)

Hence, the determinants of flow are the blood pressure within a vessel (see above) and the resistance to flow within the vessel (see below).

Velocity of blood flow

The velocity of blood flow is inversely related to the total cross-sectional area (Fig. 3.30). The branching nature of the circulatory system means that the total cross-sectional area of the capillaries is much greater than that of the arteries or veins. This substantially reduces velocity in the capillaries, allowing transport to take place.

Vascular resistance

Poiseuille's law

Poiseuille determined that resistance (R) to the steady laminar flow of a fluid through a tube is proportional to the length of the tube (l), viscosity of the fluid (η), and inversely proportional to the fourth power of the radius of the tube (r^4). He stated:

$$R = 8\eta l / \pi r^4$$

Using Ohm's law (I = V/R) we can derive:

$$\text{Flow} = (\text{Pressure difference}) \times \pi r^4 / 8 \eta l$$

From these equations we can explain the resistance element of Fig. 3.29:

- Total resistance in the vasculature is greatest in the arterioles, through a combination of their length and reduced radius without a significant change in total cross-sectional area.
- Capillary resistance is less than arteriolar resistance because capillaries are shorter (0.5 mm), large numbers of capillaries occur in parallel, and they have single-file flow rather than laminar flow.
- Total resistance is dependent upon smooth muscle tension, which controls the arteriolar radius.

Vasoconstriction and vasodilatation

Constriction of the vascular smooth muscle will cause an arteriole to narrow. This is termed vasoconstriction. Vasodilatation is the term used when smooth muscle relaxes and expands the lumen of the vessel. Vasodilatation will increase the radius of the vessel and lower its resistance. This will increase blood flow through it. Vasoconstriction will have the opposite effect, narrowing the vessel, increasing resistance, and decreasing blood flow.

Laplace's law states that the tension in the wall of a vessel needed to restore a drop in pressure across its wall is dependent upon the radius of the vessel. Or, at a given blood pressure, the tension in the wall fibres increases with the radius. Conversely, at a given radius, the tension increases with blood pressure.

This helps to explain vasoconstriction and vasodilatation. There are two components to wall tension:

- Active tension (from the vascular smooth muscle).
- Passive tension (from surrounding connective tissue – collagen and elastin).

Constriction of the smooth muscle increases active tension and decreases the radius. Assuming that the blood pressure remains constant, Laplace's law states that the net wall tension must decrease. This decrease is brought about by a fall in passive tension. That is, an equilibrium is reached between active tension, passive tension, and the internal distending pressure of the blood.

Variations in this tension bring about vasoconstriction and vasodilatation.

Blood viscosity

Viscosity, defined as 'lack of slipperiness' by Newton, is the measure of the internal friction within a moving fluid. According to Poiseuille's law, resistance is proportional to viscosity. So, viscosity of the blood plays a major role in determining resistance and, therefore, blood flow.

Plasma viscosity is increased by the presence of proteins (mainly albumins and globulins). Blood viscosity is affected by plasma viscosity, but it is the haematocrit (the percentage of red cells in the blood volume) that is the main determinant.

Haematocrit is at an optimal level for oxygen delivery. An elevated haematocrit increases the carriage of oxygen, but it raises viscosity, impeding flow and increasing cardiac work.

A normal haematocrit value of 47% makes blood viscosity about four times that of water, as measured in a special wide-bore viscometer. However, viscosity in vivo is affected by the radius of the vessels and the flow rate.

Viscosity is also affected by physiological or pathological processes, such as polycythaemia (raised haematocrit) or myeloma (cancer of immunoglobulin-secreting cells).

Polycythaemia is caused by a physiological adaptation to chronic hypoxia or a myeloproliferative disease resulting in increased red blood cell production by the bone marrow (polycythaemia rubra vera). Viscosity and, therefore, resistance are increased, leading to hypertension and sluggish blood flow.

In myeloma, there is an increased production of immunoglobulin. Immunoglobulins can cause red blood cells to agglutinate, which leads to increased blood viscosity and increased resistance. This impairs perfusion, especially in cold fingers and toes, and ischaemia/necrosis can result.

Haemodynamics of veins

Venules and veins are thin-walled, distensible vessels. They are capacitance vessels, being a variable reservoir of blood for cardiac filling. Venous blood volume depends on the venous pressure and the active wall tension (Fig. 3.31).

Active tension of the smooth muscle is controlled by sympathetic nervous stimulation, which causes venoconstriction. This pushes blood into the thoracic compartment – an important process in regulating cardiac filling pressure.

Venous pressures when supine (i.e. at heart level) are:

- 12–20 mmHg in venules.
- 8–10 mmHg in the femoral vein.
- 0–6 mmHg in the central veins and right atrium.

Although these pressures are small, resistance is also small, and the pressure is sufficient to drive blood into the right atrium.

Effect of posture and gravity

Orthostasis (the movement from supine to standing) increases blood pressure in any vessel below heart level. This is caused by the effect of gravity on the column of blood in the vessel.

Blood is prevented from flowing backwards in the veins because of the closure of venous valves. Pressure rises in the veins because blood is continually flowing into the veins from the capillaries. This will open the valves and re-establish a continuous column of blood to the heart. This means that the venous pressure in the legs increases up to 10-fold. The pressure increase will distend the venous walls and cause venous pooling in the legs. This pooling causes a fall in central venous pressure and, therefore, cardiac filling and stroke volume. Reflex mechanisms then operate, causing vasoconstriction in an attempt to maintain blood pressure.

In veins close to the right atrium, pressure becomes pulsatile. The pulse pressure in veins is not palpable, being small, but it is sufficient to distend the skin. This oscillation in pressure and, therefore, flow is caused by the motion of the heart and atrial activity (see Chapter 2 for more details). Venous flow in the great veins is also aided by the skeletal muscle pump and respiration.

Skeletal muscle pump

Rhythmic exercise, especially of the leg muscles, produces a pumping effect resulting in redistribution of venous blood into the central veins, maintaining central venous pressure (Fig. 3.32). This exercise also lowers distal venous pressure, producing an increased arteriovenous pressure difference, driving more blood into the working muscle; it also decreases capillary filtration pressure, thereby reducing swelling.

Incompetent venous valves will make the skeletal muscle pump ineffective. This means that the vertical column of blood is uninterrupted, which leads to a constant distending pressure. Permanent distension (varicose veins) may result.

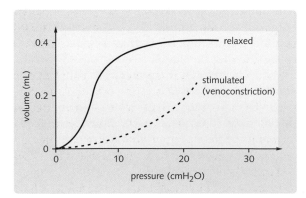

Fig. 3.31 Venous pressure curve. For a given pressure venous blood volume is greater when the venous wall muscle is relaxed than when the veins are constricted. Changes in the active wall tension can be used to displace blood into the heart.

Varicose veins are superficial tortuous dilatations of veins, usually on the legs, which frequently occur as a result of a genetic predisposition, prolonged standing, or deep venous thrombosis. They are caused by incompetent valves which allow blood to flow backwards from the deep veins of the legs to the superficial veins. They are commonly treated with surgery whereby the incompetent vein is tied, and the dilated vein stripped and removed.

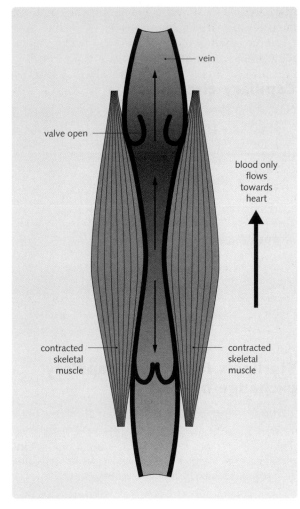

Fig. 3.32 Skeletal muscle pump. Contraction of the surrounding muscle drives the blood towards the heart. It is prevented from returning by the closure of venous valves.

Respiratory pump

In the central veins, venous return increases during inspiration. There is a fall in intrathoracic pressure, and the diaphragm compresses the abdomen, increasing abdominal pressure. The result is a rise in blood flow from the abdomen to thorax, thus increasing venous return to the right atrium and increasing right ventricular stroke volume.

Left ventricular stroke volume, however, decreases. This is primarily because the pulmonary veins are stretched, and they have a greater capacitance during inspiration, which reduces left atrial filling. The opposite occurs during expiration.

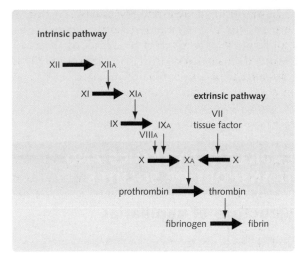

Fig. 3.33 The coagulation cascade.

Overall, the output of the two ventricles is equal over the whole respiratory cycle.

Systemic blood pressure can reflect this cycle, especially in the young. It will be:

- Decreased in inspiration.
- Increased in expiration.

Haemostasis and thrombosis

Haemostasis is the term used to refer to the regulation of blood clotting and the response of an injured vessel (i.e. vasoconstriction, see Chapter 4). It describes a dynamic balance between the maintenance of blood as a fluid and the production of a clot or thrombus at a site of injury. Note that the term thrombus is used to refer to an intravascular coagulation event, and not the physiological clot that forms when a vessel is broken open, e.g. by an external wound.

Clotting is initiated by endothelial cell injury, platelet activation, or activation of the plasma proteins (factors I–XII) which form the coagulation cascade (Fig. 3.33). The common end result is the formation of an aggregation of platelets enmeshed in cross-linked fibrin. Red and white cells may also be found in this aggregate.

Common abnormalities of haemostasis include thrombocytopenia (low platelet count) and haemophilia [heritable loss of factor VIII (A) or IX (B)] leading to slow coagulation and extensive haemorrhage. Hypercoagulable states include factor V Leiden (heritable mutation of factor V), the antiphospholipid syndrome (frequently associated with systemic lupus erythematosus) and thrombocythaemia (raised platelet count) which promote thrombus formation.

For full coverage of this subject, see *Crash Course: Immunology and Haematology* and *Crash Course: Pathology*.

CAPILLARY DYNAMICS AND TRANSPORT OF SOLUTES

Structure of capillaries

Most capillaries are thin walled, with a single layer of endothelial cells on a basement membrane. Some have a second layer of cells. There is neither smooth muscle nor elastic tissue in their walls. The arrangement of the endothelial cells determines the permeability of capillaries (see Fig. 3.20).

Laplace's law states that the tension in the wall of a vessel depends on the pressure across the wall and the radius of the vessel.

Love simplified Laplace's law, to derive an equilibrium equation that applies to a thin-walled tube:

Tension = $\Delta P \times r$

where ΔP is pressure difference and r is vessel radius.

As capillaries have very small radii, $\Delta P \times r$ will be a small value. Therefore, the tension in the wall needed to counteract the blood pressure in the capillary will be small. This, in combination with the massive total cross-sectional area, allows the capillaries to withstand blood pressure even though their walls are very thin.

Capillary circulation

Blood flow across the capillary bed is not constant but fluctuates (Fig. 3.34). Flow may be variable or even reversible – this is termed vasomotion.

Vasomotion is determined by the pathway through tissues, which is governed by the closure of different precapillary sphincters.

Arteriovenous anastomoses are not capillaries, as they contain smooth muscle. They do not undertake gaseous exchange. They are important in temperature regulation.

Capillary diameter may be smaller than red cell diameter, but because the red blood cells can deform they are still able to flow through. This may help gaseous exchange, as the cell walls are forced closer to the endothelium.

Starling's forces and capillary exchange of fluid

Starling's hypothesis of tissue fluid formation is a balance of two main forces: hydrostatic pressure (forcing fluid out of the capillaries) and osmotic pressure (also known as colloid oncotic pressure, absorbing fluid back into the capillaries).

Hydrostatic pressure results from the pressure of blood entering the capillaries from the arterioles. It is typically 37 mmHg at the arterial end of the

Fig. 3.34 Capillary circulation. Flow may be reversible in some vessels (vasomotion) depending on the closure of the precapillary sphincters.

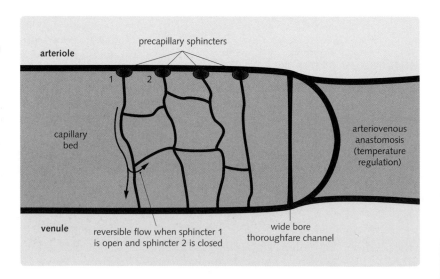

capillary and 17 mmHg at the venous end. The hydrostatic pressure of the interstitial fluid is around 0 mmHg.

Osmotic pressure is produced by the plasma proteins, as the smaller molecules can diffuse across the vessel wall equilibrating their concentrations, but large proteins cannot. Osmotic pressure in the plasma is typically 25 mmHg, and in the interstitium is 1 mmHg.

These forces balance along most of the capillary except at the two ends. At the arterial end a net filtration of fluid occurs, whereas at the venous end a net absorption takes place (Fig. 3.35). It is also probable that more filtration occurs when the precapillary sphincter is open, and more absorption occurs when the sphincter is closed.

The amount of fluid entering and leaving the capillary is small compared with the amount of fluid moving along the capillary. The exchange of fluid:

- Plays no role in the exchange of nutrients and metabolites, which occurs by diffusion.
- Is important for determining volumes of plasma and interstitial fluid.

If conditions change, the balance between filtration and absorption will change:

- An increase in hydrostatic pressure will force fluid into the interstitial space. Oedema results if there is an accumulation of fluid in this space.
- In liver disease, renal disease or severe starvation, plasma protein levels fall, decreasing osmotic pressure. This will also drive fluid into the interstitium, leading to oedema.
- Capillaries become more permeable to protein when damaged, causing a decrease in plasma osmotic pressure and leading to oedema (this process occurs, for example, in the swelling of a sprained joint).

> Capillary forces are like a seesaw. At one end, hydrostatic pressure is greater than osmotic pressure and water filters out. At the other end, osmotic pressure is greater than hydrostatic pressure and water filters in.

Capillary transport mechanisms

Exchange of solutes generally occurs by diffusion down concentration gradients. The processes involved include:

- Diffusion through the endothelial cell membrane.
- Diffusion through pores and fenestrations in the cell membrane.
- Active transportation by transcytotic vesicles (Fig. 3.36).

Lipid-soluble substances (e.g. oxygen and carbon dioxide) diffuse readily through the endothelial cell membrane of the entire capillary wall.

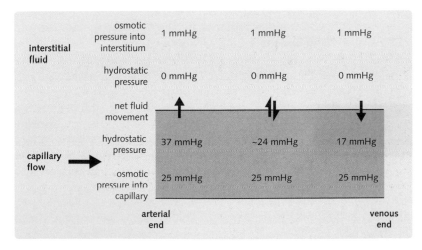

Fig. 3.35 Factors affecting fluid movement across the capillary endothelium. The fall in hydrostatic pressure across the capillary reverses the direction of fluid movement. At the arterial end, there is a net filtration pressure of $(37 - 25) - (1 - 0) = 11$ mmHg forcing fluid out of the capillary. At the venous end, this value becomes $(17 - 25) - (1 - 0) = -9$ mmHg, indicating a net filtration pressure drawing fluid back into the capillary.

Fig. 3.36 The various mechanisms of capillary transport.

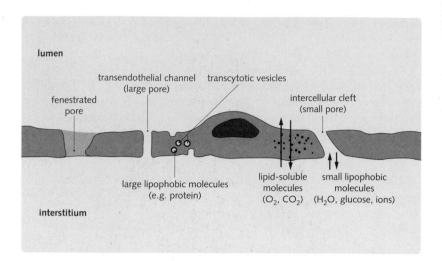

Pores and fenestrations

Water-soluble substances (e.g. water, glucose, amino acids, ions) diffuse through the many small pores (radii of 4 nm) that constitute the intercellular clefts between endothelial cells. There are also a few large pores for larger molecules, especially in the liver and spleen where the endothelium is not continuous.

Fenestrated capillaries in exocrine glands have large windows (50 nm radius), which are covered with a mesh of fibres which do not allow molecules larger than 70 kD to pass through. This makes the capillaries more permeable to water, but prevents the leakage of proteins.

In the brain, the endothelial cell junctions have a complex arrangement of fibres that make them impermeable to lipophobic molecules. This comprises the blood–brain barrier, which tightly controls the neuronal environment of the brain.

Transcytotic vesicles

Some molecules (e.g. proteins) are transported across the endothelial cell by vesicles. This is an active transport process requiring energy.

LYMPH AND THE LYMPHATIC SYSTEM

Distribution of the lymphatic tissues

Fluid and any proteins and fat globules not reabsorbed into capillaries are brought back into the blood system through the lymphatic system (Fig. 3.37). There is a network of lymphatic capillaries, ducts, and lymph nodes that unite to form the thoracic duct, which drains into the left subclavian vein.

No lymph drainage exists in the brain or eye, which have their own drainage systems – the cerebrospinal fluid and aqueous humour.

There are certain specialized areas of lymphatic tissue associated with the immune response:

- Primary lymphoid tissue – thymus and bone marrow.
- Secondary lymphoid tissue – lymph nodes, spleen, and mucosa-associated lymphoid tissue (MALT).

Further details can be found in *Crash Course: Immune, Blood, and Lymphatic Systems.*

Structure of lymph vessels

Lymph capillaries are blind ending, thin walled, and usually form a network of tubes of 10–50 μm diameter (see Fig. 3.21). These terminal lymphatics have large endothelial cell junctions, and so they are permeable to plasma proteins and other large molecules. These cell junctions may act like valves, preventing fluid moving back into the interstitium.

Lymph capillaries join together to form collecting vessels, which may contain valves to prevent backflow. Lymph vessels of this size and larger also have smooth muscle in their walls. Afferent vessels drain into a lymph node, where the fluid is presented to the immune system. Some lymph may enter the blood system at these nodes.

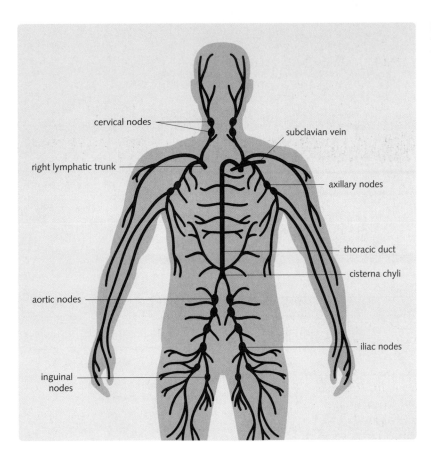

Fig. 3.37 Lymphatic drainage of the body. The lymphatics drain into the left and right subclavian veins.

cervical nodes

subclavian vein

right lymphatic trunk

axillary nodes

thoracic duct

cisterna chyli

aortic nodes

iliac nodes

inguinal nodes

Efferent vessels leave the lymph node and enter the cisterna chyli, which acts as a temporary reservoir for chylomicrons from the gut. Eventually, the lymph drains into the large thoracic duct, which drains into the left subclavian vein.

Fluid and proteins are driven into the lymphatic capillaries by the interstitial fluid pressure (possibly aided by lymphatic contraction creating suction). Lymph is moved along the lymphatics by smooth muscle contractions in the vessel wall, which increase with volume and extrinsic propulsion by the skeletal muscle pump and intestinal peristalsis. Backflow is prevented by the presence of valves.

Role of the lymphatics

The role of the lymphatic system is four-fold:

• Transportation of fluid and proteins. This maintains fluid balance by returning capillary filtrate to the blood.

• Absorption and transport of fat from the gastrointestinal tract. Chylomicrons are tiny fat globules, which are absorbed into intestinal lymph vessels (lacteals).
• Presentation of foreign materials to the immune system. Phagocytosis of particles can occur in the lymph nodes.
• Circulation of lymphocytes. If the immune response is stimulated, lymphocytes can be released from lymph nodes into the lymph to be carried into the blood.

The lymphatics are the mopping up system of the body, taking up any excess filtrate and returning it to the main circulatory system. They also carry foreign antigens from the blood to cells of the immune system located in the lymph nodes.

Control of the cardiovascular system

Objectives

You should be able to:

- List the mechanisms involved in the local control of blood flow.
- Explain how nitric oxide is involved in regulating blood flow and vessel diameter.
- Understand the mechanisms and importance of autoregulation.
- Understand the role of the autonomic nervous system in vascular control.
- Recall the effects of adrenaline, vasopressin, and the renin–angiotensin–aldosterone system on cardiovascular physiology.
- Recall the areas of the brain which influence central control.
- Recall the average flow at rest to each body system and organ.
- Explain how the Valsalva manoeuvre affects the heart and blood pressure.
- Describe the changes that occur in exercise, and understand how they are brought about.
- Understand the mechanism of vasovagal syncope.

CONTROL OF BLOOD VESSELS

Overview of vascular control

The main function of the vasculature is to deliver metabolic requirements to the tissues of the body. Some tissues have a greater need than others (Fig. 4.1), depending on their function at a given time (e.g. muscles requiring more oxygen in exercise).

Some tissues can survive without these substrates longer than others (e.g. muscle cells can survive hypoxia for hours, whereas the brain will die within minutes).

Local control mechanisms

Local temperature

The main control mechanism is in the skin. High temperature causes vasodilatation in skin arterioles and veins. In contrast, temperatures of 12–15°C cause vasoconstriction of skin vessels. This appears to be caused by noradrenergic stimulation of α_2-adrenoceptors. Below 12°C, paradoxical cold vasodilatation occurs as neurotransmitter release is impaired and vasodilator substances (e.g. prostaglandins) are released.

In most other tissues, vasodilatation occurs in response to cold. This is probably related to the predominance of α_1-receptors in other tissues compared with α_2-receptors in the skin.

Transmural pressure

This is the pressure across the wall of the vessel, and it can be affected by external and internal pressures:

- External pressure. Blood flow is impaired by a high external pressure outside the vessel (e.g. when muscle is contracted or when sitting or kneeling).
- Internal pressure. Initially, an increase in blood pressure causes the vessels to distend briefly. This causes the smooth muscle to be stretched, producing a contracting response. The vessel becomes constricted, increasing resistance and reducing flow within the vessel. This is termed the 'myogenic response', and is a mechanism of autoregulation.

Local metabolites

Altered levels of many metabolites cause vasodilatation and increase perfusion of the tissue. These include:

- Hypoxia (i.e. decreased P_{O_2}).
- Acidosis (caused by CO_2 and/or lactate).

Distribution of cardiac output				
Organ	Mass (kg)	Blood flow (mL/min)	Blood flow per 100 g (mL/min/100 g)	Proportion of cardiac output (%)
Brain	1.4	750	54.0	13.9 [18.4]
Heart	0.3	250	84.0	4.7 [11.6]
Liver	1.5	1500*	100.0*	27.8 [20.4]*
(Gastrointestinal tract)	(2.5)	(1170)	(46.8)	(21.7 [16.0])
Kidneys	0.3	1260	420	23.3 [7.2]
Skeletal muscle	31.0	840	2.7	15.6 [20.0]
Skin	3.6	460	12.8	8.6 [4.8]
Rest of body	22.4	340	1.5	6.1 [17.6]
Whole body	63.0	5400	8.6	100 [100]

Fig. 4.1 Distribution of cardiac output to the various systems of the body. Note that the blood flow to the gastrointestinal tract (shown in round brackets) also flows through the liver via the portal circulation. Values for the liver marked * include the portal and arterial circulation to the liver. Values in square brackets denote the percentage of oxygen consumption by the various systems.

- Adenosine triphosphate (ATP) breakdown products.
- K^+ (from contracting muscle and active brain neurons).
- Increase in osmolarity.

Different tissues are influenced to varying degrees by these factors; e.g. coronary vessels react mainly to hypoxia and adenosine whereas cerebral vessels are influenced by K^+, H^+, and P_{CO_2}.

Most locally produced substances increase blood flow because the tissue wants to wash them away (e.g. lactate and adenosine are waste products of metabolism, which need to be removed).

Cytokines

Cytokines are chemical substances that are produced, secreted and act locally as hormones producing focal responses (e.g. inflammation, haemorrhage). They include:

- Histamine. This is an inflammatory mediator that causes arteriolar vasodilatation (H_1 receptor mediated). In veins, it causes vasoconstriction and increased permeability (H_2 receptor mediated).
- Bradykinin. This inflammatory mediator causes endothelium-dependent vasodilatation and increases vascular permeability.
- 5-Hydroxytryptamine (5-HT, serotonin). This is found in platelets, the intestinal wall, and the central nervous system. It causes vasoconstriction. Production from platelets contributes significantly to vasoconstriction in response to vessel injury.
- Prostaglandins (PGs). These are inflammatory mediators synthesized from arachidonic acid by cyclo-oxygenase (COX). They are produced by macrophages, leucocytes, fibroblasts, and endothelium. Their production is inhibited by non-steroidal anti-inflammatory drugs (NSAIDs) and steroids. PGF causes vasoconstriction; PGE and PGI_2 (prostacyclin) cause vasodilatation.
- Thromboxane A_2. This is a platelet activator that causes vasoconstriction; it is involved in haemostasis.

- Leukotrienes. These are inflammatory mediators synthesized from arachidonic acid by lipoxygenase. They are produced by leucocytes, and cause vasoconstriction and increased vascular permeability.
- Platelet activating factor (PAF). This is an inflammatory mediator that causes vasodilatation, increased vascular permeability, and vasospasm in hypoxic coronary vessels.

Endothelium-dependent relaxation and contraction

When stimulated, the endothelium of arteries and veins produce endothelium-derived relaxing factor (EDRF), later discovered to be nitric oxide (NO). Stimuli for its secretion include thrombin, bradykinin, substance-P, adenosine diphosphate (ADP), acetylcholine, and histamine.

NO diffuses into smooth muscle cells and activates an intracellular cyclic guanosine monophosphate (cGMP) messenger system, causing relaxation and vasodilatation.

The products of platelet activation stimulate NO release from intact endothelium to ensure that vasoconstriction only occurs with significant endothelial damage. Healthy endothelium will maintain vessel patency through NO, while injured endothelium will not counteract platelet-initiated vasoconstriction.

Blood flowing through an artery causes shear stress on the endothelial cell. When arterioles dilate to increase tissue perfusion, flow increases in feeder arteries by a process called flow-induced vasodilatation. This process is caused by increased shear stress, increasing NO production.

Vasoconstrictor substances are also produced by the endothelium – prostanoid is produced in large arteries to cause constriction in response to hypoxia; endothelin is a powerful vasoconstrictive peptide released in response to stretch, thrombin, and adrenaline. Endothelin acts locally, but it seems to have a role in the systemic regulation of blood pressure, and it has been the target for experimental therapeutic agents in the pulmonary circulation.

Autoregulation and hyperaemia

Autoregulation is the process whereby tissue perfusion remains relatively constant even though blood pressure changes. It also keeps capillary filtration pressure at a stable value.

Flow is proportional to (pressure difference)/resistance. Therefore, to keep flow constant, any pressure change must be opposed by a resistance change. An increase in pressure causes arteriolar vasoconstriction, thereby increasing resistance. A decrease in pressure causes arteriolar vasodilatation and decreases resistance. It takes 30–60 s for the effect to take place so, for example, there is an initial increase in flow with a pressure increase before a steady state is reached.

Autoregulation only occurs over a limited pressure range. It is an intrinsic feature of the vessels, and it is independent of nervous control. However, it does not mean that tissue perfusion is constant all the time in vivo. Autoregulation can be reset to work at a new level by, for example, an increased sympathetic drive. The mechanisms for autoregulation are:

- Myogenic response. Increased pressure produces constriction of the vessel, opposing the rise in pressure and stabilizing blood flow.
- Vasodilator washout. This is the effect that blood flow has on the concentration of the local vasodilator metabolites. If blood flow increases, these metabolites are washed away faster, causing the vessel to constrict, thereby increasing resistance and slowing flow.
- In the heart any increase in coronary arterial pressure causes a rise in tissue P_{O_2}, leading to vasoconstriction; this autoregulates heart blood flow.

Metabolic hyperaemia

Metabolic (or functional/active) hyperaemia is the increase in blood flow that occurs in exercising muscle and secreting exocrine glands when their metabolic rate increases. The production of local vasodilator metabolites leads to vasodilatation and causes vascular resistance to fall.

Flow-induced vasodilatation causes the main artery to dilate. Ascending dilatation from the arterioles to the feeder arteries leads to dilatation of the whole arterial tree supplying the tissue.

Blood flow in contracting muscle is increased in the resting phase. In the heart, the increase in metabolic rate causes a drop in tissue P_{O_2}, leading to vasodilatation.

Reactive hyperaemia

Reactive (or post-ischaemic) hyperaemia is the increase in blood flow that occurs after supply to a tissue has been temporarily interrupted.

Reactive hyperaemia enables resupply to ischaemic tissue as quickly as possible. The myogenic response is the predominant mechanism for brief occlusions, dilating the downstream vessels in preparation for the return of blood flow. In more prolonged occlusions, vasodilator metabolites accumulate, and these play a significant role. Prostaglandins also aid this process.

Reactive hyperaemia is temporary, and it decays exponentially. A plateau of hyperaemia may precede decay in prolonged occlusions. In some tissues (e.g. the heart), there is oversupply of blood and oxygen compared with the deficit during the temporary interruption to flow.

Ischaemic reperfusion injury

When blood flow to a tissue is interrupted for a prolonged period, reactive hyperaemia is impaired.

Reperfusion of ischaemic tissue results in superoxide ($O_2^{-\bullet}$) and hydroxide ($OH^\bullet$) radical formation. These damage the tissue and vessel wall, causing further occlusion. Damage is exacerbated by an increase in K^+ and tissue acidosis. Reperfused cells have an impaired barrier to Ca^{2+} ions, which flow into the cell in an unrestricted way, causing calcium overload and subsequent damage.

It is thought that reperfusion injury exacerbates damage to the myocardium, intestine and brain following ischaemia.

> Patients with crush injuries are an uncommon occurrence, but nonetheless doctors should be prepared to deal with them. Standard advice to first aiders is that if a casualty has a part of their body crushed, and the object has been there for more than 10 minutes, then the possibility of allowing toxic metabolites from the trapped segment to enter the systemic circulation when the object is removed is significant.

Nervous control

Fig. 4.2 gives an overview of nervous control of the vasculature.

Sympathetic vasoconstrictor nerves

Sympathetic vasoconstrictor nerves innervate the vascular smooth muscle of the resistance and capacitance vessels. A basal level of activity of these nerves is responsible for vessel tone at rest. The neurotransmitter involved is noradrenaline, which acts on α_1-receptors on vascular smooth muscle causing contraction. When there is an increase in sympathetic drive:

- Vasoconstriction decreases local blood flow.
- Venoconstriction decreases local blood volume.
- Arteriolar constriction decreases capillary pressure, leading to greater resorption of fluid from the interstitium back into the blood.

If there is an increase in sympathetic activity throughout the body, total peripheral resistance and cardiac output increase. This constitutes the basis of the sympathetic response to haemorrhage.

A decrease in sympathetic activity causes vasodilatation and venodilatation.

Sympathetic vasodilator nerves

Some tissues (skeletal muscle and sweat glands) are also innervated by sympathetic vasodilator nerves.

In skeletal muscle, vascular bed stimulation by these nerves (which use acetylcholine as the neurotransmitter and act on muscarinic receptors) causes vasodilatation. Stimulation only occurs as part of an 'alerting response', and it is initiated in the forebrain without any brainstem influence. The vasodilator effect is only temporary, and it plays no role in blood pressure regulation. Stimulation of these nerves in sweat glands – probably involving vasoactive intestinal peptide (VIP) as neurotransmitter – produces sweating and cutaneous vasodilatation.

Parasympathetic vasodilator nerves

Parasympathetic vasodilator nerves innervate the blood vessels of the:

- Head and neck.
- Salivary glands.
- Pancreas.
- Gastrointestinal mucosa.
- Genitalia.
- Bladder.

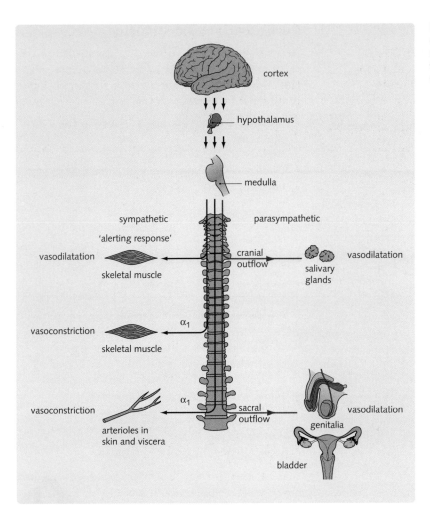

Fig. 4.2 Overview of nervous control of the vasculature. The sympathetic tracts are shown on the left and the parasympathetic tracts on the right.

The effect of these nerves on the total peripheral resistance is small because of their limited innervation. Their postganglionic neurons release acetylcholine, which relaxes vascular smooth muscle.

In some tissues (e.g. the pancreas), VIP may be the main neurotransmitter. Vasodilatation occurs in the arteries and arterioles of these vascular beds.

In the erectile tissue of the penis, it is parasympathetic and nitrergic vasodilatation (see below) that fills the corpus sinuses with blood, causing erection.

Nitrergic vasodilator nerves

Nitric oxide is a recognized neurotransmitter, both in the central and peripheral nervous system. The neurons upon which it acts are referred to as nitrergic. They act on smooth muscle cells, causing relaxation. Nitrergic innervation has so far been found in the regulation of muscle tone in the gut and in sexual arousal in the male and female genitalia.

At present, pharmacological manipulation of nitrergic transmission is limited to the use of sildenafil (Viagra) in the treatment of male impotence. Sildenafil acts by selective inhibition of the phosphodiesterase present in smooth muscle of the genital vessels. This potentiates the effect of nitrergic stimulation (phosphodiesterase enzymes break up the cGMP that mediates the relaxation in response to NO). Sildenafil should not be given to hypotensive patients, nor combined with other forms of systemic nitrate treatment due to the risk of syncope.

Hormonal control

Although the vasculature is influenced by circulating hormones, short-term control is mainly achieved by the nervous system. Further details of these hormones can be found in *Crash Course: Endocrine and Reproductive Systems*.

Adrenaline

The catecholamines (adrenaline and noradrenaline) are secreted from the adrenal medulla.

More than three times as much adrenaline is secreted as noradrenaline. Plasma levels at rest of adrenaline are 0.1–0.5 nmol/L, and noradrenaline 0.5–3.0 nmol/L. There is more noradrenaline in plasma because of spill-over from sympathetic nerve terminals. Secretion is increased in exercise, hypotension, hypoglycaemia, and 'fight or flight' situations. It is also important to remember that there are adrenoceptors present on non-cardiac sites, such as β-adrenoceptors on the smooth muscle of the airway.

Both hormones are β-adrenoceptor agonists, so they increase heart rate and contractility of the myocardium (see p. 17). Both hormones cause vasoconstriction in most tissues via α-receptors:

- Adrenaline causes vasoconstriction in most organs (especially skin), but vasodilatation in skeletal muscle, myocardium, and liver. This is because there are more β-receptors in these latter tissues, and adrenaline has a higher affinity for these receptors.
- Noradrenaline usually causes vasoconstriction because it has a higher affinity for α-receptors.

Adrenal gland stimulation results predominantly in adrenaline release. Effects on the heart include increased contractility, stroke volume, and heart rate. Blood pressure rises as a result, since the vasodilatory effects of adrenaline do not fully counteract the vasoconstrictor effects combined with the increased cardiac output.

Vasopressin (antidiuretic hormone)

Antidiuretic hormone (ADH) is a peptide produced in the hypothalamus and released from the posterior pituitary directly into the bloodstream. A rise in plasma osmolarity is the main stimulus for secretion. Falling blood pressure and volume are also stimuli, but to a lesser degree.

ADH promotes water retention by the kidney by opening channels predominantly sited in the collecting ducts. High levels of ADH also cause vasoconstriction in most tissues. In the brain and heart, NO-mediated vasodilatation occurs ensuring preferential supply in hypovolaemic states.

Renin–angiotensin–aldosterone

Renin is an enzyme produced by the juxtaglomerular cells of the kidney. It converts angiotensinogen (from the liver) to angiotensin I (Fig. 4.3). Renin production is increased by:

- A fall in afferent arterial pressure to the glomeruli.
- Increased sympathetic activity.
- Decreased Na^+ in the macula densa of the adjacent tubule.

Angiotensin-converting enzyme (ACE) converts angiotensin I to the peptide angiotensin II (Fig. 4.3), predominantly in the pulmonary vascular bed. It has the following actions:

- Increases aldosterone secretion from the adrenal cortex.
- Causes vasoconstriction at high concentration by acting directly on vascular smooth muscle, initiating release of noradrenaline from sympathetic nerve terminals, and increasing central sympathetic drive in the brainstem.
- Increases cardiac contractility.

Aldosterone increases Na^+ and therefore water retention in the distal convoluted tubule, at the expense of excreting K^+.

It is important to remember that renin and ACE are enzymes, angiotensinogen and angiotensin I are substrates, angiotensin II causes independent vasoconstriction and stimulates aldosterone production.

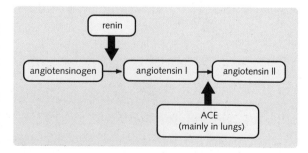

Fig. 4.3 Formation of angiotensin II. Angiotensinogen is secreted by the liver, acted on by renin (secreted by the kidney) and finally converted to the active angiotensin II by angiotensin-converting enzyme (ACE).

Atrial and brain natriuretic peptides

In response to high cardiac filling pressure, specialized myocytes in the atria secrete atrial natriuretic peptide (ANP). ANP increases the excretion of salt and water by renal tubules. It also has a small vasodilating effect.

Ventricles similarly secrete brain natriuretic peptide (BNP), which increases in heart failure. BNP levels may be assayed to test for heart failure.

CARDIOVASCULAR RECEPTORS AND CENTRAL CONTROL

The cardiovascular system is ultimately regulated and controlled by the brain through autonomic nerves (Fig. 4.4).

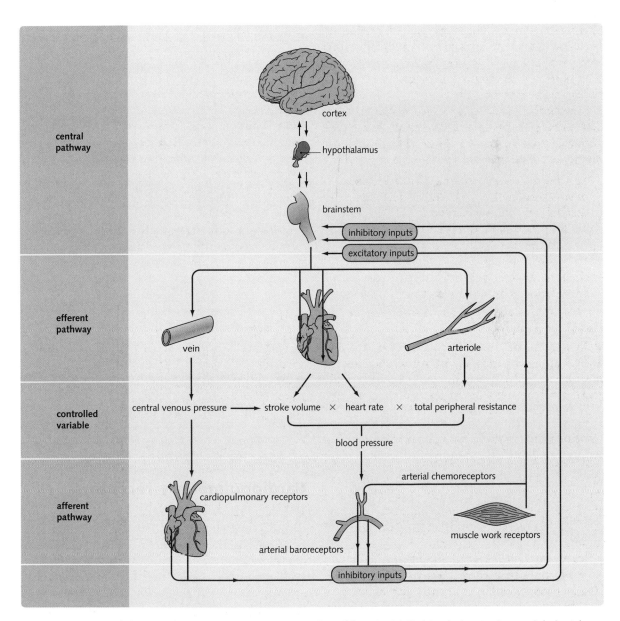

Fig. 4.4 Overview of the central control of the circulation. (Adapted from Levick R. Introducing cardiovascular physiology. London: Butterworth-Heinemann, 1995. Reproduced by permission of Edward Arnold Ltd.)

Arterial baroreceptors and the baroreflex

Arterial baroreceptors (stretch receptors) are located in the carotid sinus and aortic arch. They play a key role in short-term blood pressure control, and they respond to stretch of the vessel wall. They continually produce impulses at normal vessel wall tone. Increased stretch (due to increased pressure) increases firing frequency, whereas decreased stretch decreases the firing rate.

The impulse that the baroreceptor generates is carried to the medulla by the glossopharyngeal nerves (carotid sinus) and the vagus nerves (aortic arch).

A 34-year-old pregnant lady comes into hospital with palpitations and shortness of breath. The ECG monitor shows a supraventricular tachycardia, although the exact rhythm cannot be seen. Carotid sinus massage, Valsalva manoeuvre and eliciting the diving reflex would all be sensible first-line treatments to lower the heart rate before resorting to drugs such as adenosine. Massaging of the carotid sinus stimulates the baroreceptor present there.

At the medulla, there is an interaction with the other central pathways. An increased firing rate causes the medulla to:

- Increase vagal (parasympathetic) drive.
- Decrease sympathetic drive.

This results in a decrease in heart rate. Contractility is probably not affected. It also causes a fall in total peripheral resistance. These measures all serve to reduce blood pressure back to normal. The baroreceptors are said to buffer the blood pressure in the short term.

When the baroreceptor is unloaded (stretch is reduced), the firing rate to the medulla is reduced. The effect is to decrease vagal and increase sympathetic drive. This results in:

- Increased heart rate and contractility.
- Peripheral vasoconstriction and venoconstriction.
- Catecholamine secretion.
- Increased renin secretion.

The effect is to increase cardiac output, total peripheral resistance, and the circulating volume, all of which serve to return blood pressure to normal.

The baroreflex is very rapid (<1 s for bradycardia to occur), and it is very important in acute hypotension and haemorrhage.

The sensitivity of the arterial baroreceptors to a change in blood pressure is decreased by:

- Age. The compliance of the arterial wall falls with age, which means there is less stretch of the arterial walls.
- Chronic hypertension. The arterial wall loses its distensibility.

The baroreflex is inhibited by stimulation of the hypothalamic defence area in 'fight or flight' situations.

The level of blood pressure that the baroreceptor takes as normal (the setting or set point) can be reset by central or peripheral processes:

- Central resetting. In exercise, the rise in blood pressure that occurs does not cause a bradycardia because there has been a central influence to operate the baroreflex at a new higher level. The neurons that drive inspiration inhibit cardiac vagal nerves, so blocking baroreceptor impulses and causing a decreased vagal drive. This explains the increased heart rate with inspiration (sinus arrhythmia).
- Peripheral resetting. Chronic hyper- or hypotension leads to the set point being reset to this new pressure, thus allowing the baroreflex to operate in its optimal range. This is also the reason why the baroreflex is not very useful for long-term blood pressure homeostasis, and why the rapid lowering of blood pressure in patients with longstanding hypertension is potentially very dangerous.

Cardiopulmonary receptors

There are many cardiopulmonary receptors connected to afferent fibres innervating the heart, great veins, and pulmonary artery. Overall, stimulation of these receptors causes bradycardia, vasodilatation and hypotension. There are three main classes of receptor with differing functions – venoatrial stretch receptors, unmyelinated mechanoreceptor fibres, and chemosensitive fibres.

Venoatrial stretch receptors

These are branched nerve endings located where the great veins join the atria. They are connected to large myelinated vagal fibres. Stimulation produces a reflex tachycardia by selectively increasing sympathetic drive to the pacemaker. There is also an increase in salt and water excretion.

Unmyelinated mechanoreceptor fibres

These are present in both atria and in the left ventricle. Afferent fibres travel in vagal and sympathetic nerves. Large distension stimulates these receptors, causing an inhibitory effect. Reflex bradycardia and peripheral vasodilatation occurs.

Chemosensitive fibres

Some unmyelinated vagal and sympathetic afferents are chemosensitive. They are stimulated in response to bradykinin and other substances released by an ischaemic myocardium. It is thought that the pain of angina and myocardial infarction are caused by these fibres. Stimulation increases respiration as well as causing bradycardia and peripheral vasodilatation.

Other excitatory inputs

Arterial chemoreceptors

Chemoreceptors are located in the carotid and aortic bodies. They are nerve terminals whose excitation is increased by hypoxia, hypercapnia, and acidosis of arterial blood (see *Crash Course: Respiratory System*). Their fibres travel with afferent baroreceptor fibres in the glossopharyngeal and vagus nerves.

At normal gas tensions, chemoreceptors are mainly involved in the control of breathing. However, when their excitation is increased, they respond by causing a sympathetically mediated vasoconstriction and a mild bradycardia. The respiratory chemoreflex increases tidal volume, which stimulates lung stretch receptors. This causes a marked tachycardia and a modest vasodilatation. Overall, the heart rate and blood pressure increase to enhance perfusion. The chemoreflex plays an important role in asphyxia, severe haemorrhage, and hypotension, where the chemoreceptors are excited by the reduced metabolite supply (and blood pressure is below baroreceptor range).

Muscle receptors

Skeletal muscle produces a reflex cardiovascular response to exercise. This is stimulated by metaboloreceptors (activated by K^+ and H^+) and mechanoreceptors (activated by pressure and tension). The excitation travels through small nerve fibres (groups III and IV). The reflex produces tachycardia, increased myocardial contractility, and vasoconstriction in other vascular beds. This allows greater perfusion of the exercising muscle, and is termed the exercise pressor response.

Central pathways

The central pathways that influence the cardiovascular system have only been partly explained. They involve a complex interaction between the medulla, hypothalamus, cerebellum, and cortex.

Medulla

It used to be thought that there was a specific vasomotor centre in the medulla. Now, it is thought that there are complex signals between the hypothalamus, cortex, and cerebellum as well as signals within the vasomotor centre of the medulla. The rostral ventrolateral medulla is responsible for the sympathetic outflow, whereas the nucleus ambiguus is responsible for the parasympathetic outflow; these two areas control vessel tone and heart rate.

Information from baroreceptors is received (at the nucleus tractus solitarius) by the medulla, and it is relayed to the hypothalamus. Medullary autonomic control is also influenced by hypothalamic activity.

Hypothalamus

This contains four areas of interest:

- Depressor area. This can produce the baroreflex, but it is not vital for the reflex to occur.
- Defence area. This is responsible for the alerting response and the 'fight or flight' response, thus playing a role in governing sympathetic outflow.
- Temperature-regulating area. This controls cutaneous vascular tone and sweating.
- Vasopressin-secreting area. This produces vasopressin, which travels through nerve axons to the pituitary.

Cerebellum

The cerebellum's primary role is muscle coordination. During exercise, the cerebellum helps to coordinate the response to exercise.

Cortex

The cortex may initiate many of the cardiovascular responses. The effects of fear and emotion on the vasculature probably have a cortical influence.

REGULATION OF CIRCULATION IN INDIVIDUAL TISSUES

Blood flow rates in various circulations are given in Fig. 4.5.

Coronary circulation

Myocardial oxygen demand is very high, being about 8 ml O_2/min/100 g. During exercise, cardiac work can increase five-fold, thereby increasing oxygen demand. Oxygen levels in coronary venous blood are very low, so demand can only be met by increasing arterial flow.

Oxygen transport is aided by the high capillary density (large area and decreased distance for exchange) and the presence of myoglobin. There is a high oxygen extraction from the capillaries (>60%) even at rest.

Blood flow is mainly controlled by tissue P_{O_2}. Low P_{O_2} produces a metabolic hyperaemia. Metabolic vasodilatation can be partly opposed by sympathetic α_1-noradrenergic vasoconstriction. Adrenaline acts on β_2-receptors in coronary smooth muscle to dilate the vessels.

Coronary arteries are functional end-arteries with few cross-connections between them. They are at risk of being blocked by thrombosis, causing ischaemia. There are, however, some collateral vessels which may delay the onset of ischaemia. During systole, coronary artery branches in the myocardium are compressed. Flow is fully restored only during diastole (Fig. 4.6).

Skeletal muscle

Oxygen and nutrient delivery to the muscle cells must increase with exercise. Removal of waste products and heat must also be increased during exercise.

Physically active muscle consists of white fibres (e.g. gastrocnemius). Postural muscles (e.g. soleus) are tonically active red fibres, and they have a greater capillary density.

Sympathetic vasoconstrictor nerve reflexes controlled by baroreceptors play a major role in controlling flow. In hypovolaemia, for example, vasoconstriction can reduce flow in skeletal muscle to one-fifth of its resting value.

Flow rate in various circulations		
Circulation	Basal flow rate (mL/min/100 g)	Maximum flow rate (minimum) (mL/min/100 g)
Coronary	80	400
Phasic (white, fast) skeletal muscle	3	200 (on exercise)
Tonic (red, slow) skeletal muscle	15	200 (on exercise)
Cutaneous	10–20 (at 27°C)	200
Brain Grey matter	55 100	— —
Renal	400	—
Liver GIT	85 40	150 (after food) 80 (after food)

Fig. 4.5 Resting and maximum blood flow rates in the various circulations (GIT, gastrointestinal tract).

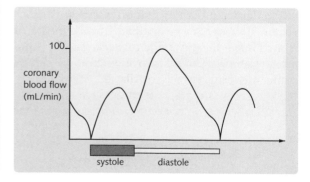

Fig. 4.6 Coronary blood flow during the cardiac cycle. Note that maximal blood flow is during diastole.

Skeletal muscle makes up 40% of body mass. Its vasculature contributes significantly to vascular resistance and, therefore, affects blood pressure homeostasis.

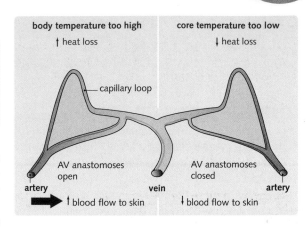

Fig. 4.7 Temperature control by arteriovenous (AV) anastomoses.

During exercise, metabolic vasodilatation is the dominant mechanism for increasing flow. Adrenaline causes vasodilatation by acting on smooth-muscle β_2-receptors.

At rest, only 25% of the oxygen in the blood is extracted. In severe exercise, this extraction can be increased considerably. Extraction is aided by the presence of myoglobin.

The skeletal muscle pump aids venous return to the heart. This lowers venous pressure in the limbs, hence increasing the pressure difference from the arterial to venous circulation. Perfusion pressure therefore increases, driving blood flow.

Blood flow is impaired during contraction. If contraction is sustained then the fibres will become hypoxic. Lactate will accumulate causing pain, and strength will be rapidly lost.

Cutaneous circulation

The skin has a low metabolic requirement, and its vasculature is mainly involved in the regulation of the internal core body temperature.

Specific areas of the skin have arteriovenous anastomoses (Fig. 4.7). These exposed areas have a high surface area to volume ratio and include the fingers, toes, palms, soles of the feet, lips, nose, and ears. These anastomoses are controlled by sympathetic vasoconstrictor nerves. In turn the sympathetic activity is controlled via the brainstem by the temperature-regulating area in the hypothalamus. The nerves controlling sweating are also controlled in the same way – when the core body temperature is too high, sympathetic drive is reduced and the arteriovenous anastomoses dilate.

Skin temperature is very variable as it is influenced by ambient temperature. It has a direct effect on cutaneous vascular tone:

- Local heating causes vasodilatation.
- Local cooling causes vasoconstriction.

Paradoxical cold vasodilatation occurs in acral areas (the extremities) on prolonged exposure to cold. After the initial vasoconstriction, vasodilatation occurs. This is thought to be because the cold impairs sympathetic vasoconstriction.

Hypotension causes a neural and hormonal (angiotensin, ADH and adrenaline) vasoconstriction of skin vessels. This produces the cold skin seen in shock.

Exercise causes vasoconstriction of the skin initially, but this can become a dilatation if the core temperature rises.

Emotion can produce a hyperaemic response in the skin (blushing) and the gastric and colonic mucosa.

Compression of the skin for long periods (e.g. when sitting) impairs blood flow. Reactive hyperaemia and the skin's high tolerance to hypoxia prevents ischaemic damage. Restlessness (i.e. the desire to move position) also plays a major role, possibly stimulated by local metabolites and pain receptors. In certain patients, however, failure to move or be moved can lead to necrosis in compressed areas (pressure sores).

In hot weather, cutaneous vasodilatation can lower central venous pressure. This can lead to fainting, for example when soldiers stand on a hot day, they must use their muscle pumps to maintain venous return from their legs.

Cerebral circulation

Grey matter has a high oxygen consumption (7 mL O_2/min/100 g). As grey matter has little tolerance to hypoxia, consciousness is lost after a few seconds of ischaemia.

The main function of the cardiovascular system is to maintain an adequate supply of oxygen to the brain. The cerebral circulation can adjust itself locally to meet local demand. This is mainly by an increase in interstitial K^+, causing metabolic hyperaemia.

In young people, the circle of Willis enables blood supply to be maintained if one carotid artery is occluded. These anastomoses linking the supply arteries together are less effective in the elderly. There is a high capillary density, similar in size to that in the myocardium. The presence of a blood–brain barrier tightly controls the neuronal environment. Lipid-soluble molecules can diffuse freely, but ionic solutes cannot.

The brain can control cardiac output and vascular resistance of other tissues through autonomic nerves. Cerebral perfusion is maintained at the expense of other tissues when required.

There is good autoregulation of the cerebral blood flow, but this eventually fails when pressure falls below 50 mmHg.

Cerebral vessels are very sensitive to arterial P_{CO_2}:

- Hypercapnia causes vasodilatation (Fig. 4.8).
- Hypocapnia causes vasoconstriction.

Reduction in arterial P_{CO_2} through hyperventilation can lead to cerebral vasoconstriction, and even transient unconsciousness. Cerebral vessels do not participate in baroreflex vasoconstriction.

> The body is very good at diverting blood flow to where it is needed.
> However, some circulations (e.g. cerebral and renal) are special in that their blood flow is usually preserved at the expense of others.

Pulmonary circulation

The entire output of the right ventricle enters the pulmonary circulation. A separate bronchial circulation from the aorta meets the metabolic needs of the bronchi.

There is a very high capillary density and very thin blood–alveolar surface to maximize gaseous exchange. Gas exchange in the lung is flow limited (i.e. a rise in blood flow increases the rate of oxygen uptake).

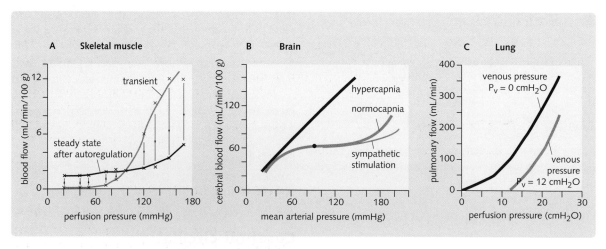

Fig. 4.8 Pressure–flow curves for (A) skeletal muscle, (B) brain vasculature and (C) lung tissue. In (A) one line shows transient flow after altering perfusion pressure; the other line shows steady state achieved by autoregulation. (B) shows autoregulation at normal arterial P_{CO_2} and the effect of hypercapnia. In (C) the airway pressure was constant at 4 cmH$_2$O. Increasing perfusion pressure increases pulmonary flow due to vascular distension and opening of some closed venous vessels. This increase in flow is less marked when venous pressure is above airway pressure.

Pulmonary arteries and arterioles are shorter, thinner walled, and more easily distensible than systemic vessels so that pulmonary vascular resistance is very low with a low pulmonary arterial pressure (22/8 mmHg). There is no autoregulation of blood flow, although the pulmonary vessels still respond to systemic mediators (e.g. adrenaline).

Low capillary pressure means that there is no filtration of fluid into the alveoli in health.

In the upright person, mean arterial pressure at the apex of the lung is about 3 mmHg and at the base is about 21 mmHg. At the level of the heart, the mean pressure is 15 mmHg. At the lung base, high pressure causes the thin-walled vessels to distend and blood flow to increase (Fig. 4.8). At the apex, flow only occurs during systole, as the diastolic pressure is insufficient to open the vessels.

The ventilation–perfusion ratio governs the efficiency of oxygen transfer. Although ventilation is greater at the base than at the apex, the difference is not as great as the difference in flow. This implies that ventilation–perfusion ratio is higher at the apex than at the base, and this mismatch impairs efficiency.

General hypoxia causes pulmonary hypertension. Poorly ventilated areas become poorly perfused because of hypoxic vasoconstriction. This mechanism helps to optimize ventilation–perfusion ratios.

Renal circulation

Renal blood flow is autoregulated over a certain range of blood pressure. This allows a near-constant glomerular filtration rate. Autoregulation fails in severe hypotension (prerenal failure).

Mesenteric circulation

The hyperaemia associated with the arrival of food is caused by:

- Local hormones (e.g. gastrin and cholecystokinin).
- Digestion products (e.g. glucose and fatty acids).
- Increased vagal activity.

The rise in mesenteric/splanchnic blood flow produces a tachycardia and, therefore, an increase in cardiac output of 1 L/min. There is also vasoconstriction in skeletal muscle vascular beds. There is normally no significant change in blood pressure.

COORDINATED CARDIOVASCULAR RESPONSES

Cardiovascular response to posture

When moving from supine to standing (orthostasis), the effect of gravity on venous blood causes venous pooling in the legs. There is a fall in intrathoracic blood volume. This leads to decreased cardiac filling and, therefore, decreased stroke volume and a fall in pressure. This is often corrected immediately by the baroreflex, but it can cause a transient hypotension, even in healthy individuals. This happens especially when there is already peripheral vasodilatation in a warm environment.

The baroreceptors and cardiopulmonary receptors react by decreasing their firing rate. This increases sympathetic outflow and decreases vagal drive, resulting in an increased heart rate (of about 20 beats/min) and contractility. Peripheral vasoconstriction increases total peripheral resistance, which helps increase blood pressure. Venoconstriction also plays a limited role in helping to reverse venous pooling. Capillary filtration in the leg increases because of the increase in venous pressure. This may cause a drop in plasma volume over time. Vasopressin and aldosterone (via renin–angiotensin) reduce salt and water excretion in order to increase plasma volume. The overall effect is a maintenance of arterial pressure and, thus, cerebral perfusion.

Failure of this mechanism causes postural hypotension, a decrease in systolic blood pressure of >15 mmHg on standing which may be associated with symptoms of light-headedness or even collapse.

Valsalva manoeuvre

This is a forced expiration against a closed glottis. This commonly occurs when coughing, defecating, and lifting heavy weights. It produces a raised intrathoracic pressure

This manoeuvre is a useful test of baroreceptor competence (Fig. 4.9). If the pressure fall in phase 2 continues and there is no bradycardia in phase 4,

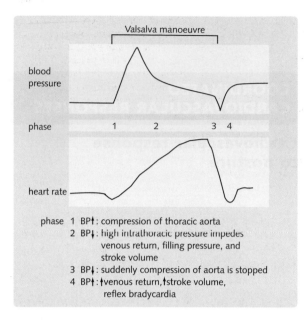

Fig. 4.9 Response to the Valsalva manoeuvre (BP, blood pressure).

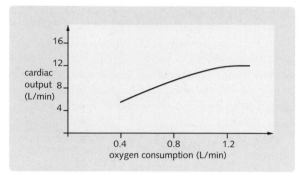

Fig. 4.10 Relationship between cardiac output and oxygen consumption in the whole body. It shows a linear increase of cardiac output with oxygen consumption produced by increased heart rate and stroke volume.

then the baroreflex is being interrupted, leading to postural hypotension.

Cardiovascular response to exercise

Initial requirements during exercise are:

- Increased gaseous exchange in the pulmonary circulation.
- Increased blood flow to the working muscle.
- Stable blood pressure.

Cardiac output and oxygen uptake

Cardiac output is increased by increases in heart rate or stroke volume (Fig. 4.10):

- Increased heart rate can be caused by sympathetic stimulation or decreased vagal inhibition.
- Stroke volume can be increased by increased cardiac filling (due to skeletal muscle pump and splanchnic vasoconstriction), increased contractility (due to sympathetic stimulation), or a fall in peripheral resistance (due to skeletal muscle vasodilatation).

In upright exercise, stroke volume plays the main role in increasing output. In supine exercise, heart rate increases mainly account for the increased output. Stroke volume increases only at low work rates.

Changes in blood flow to active muscle

Blood flow to active muscle increases with exercise. Hyperaemia can be as much as 40 times normal flow, and it is caused by:

- Metabolic vasodilatation.
- Increased pressure gradient by skeletal muscle pump in upright exercise.
- Capillary recruitment by dilatation of terminal arterioles.

The alerting response caused by anticipation of exercise (e.g. at the start of a race) causes an initial sympathetically mediated vasodilatation.

Changes in blood flow in other tissues

Coronary blood flow increases with the increase in cardiac work. Cutaneous vessels initially contract to maintain blood pressure, but dilate if core temperature rises. Vasoconstriction in the renal, splanchnic, and non-active muscle vascular beds helps to maintain blood pressure.

Blood pressure during static and dynamic exercise

In dynamic (alternately contracting and relaxing) exercise, the diastolic pressure hardly changes although the pulse pressure rises (Fig. 4.11). The increase in pressure in static exercise is caused by the

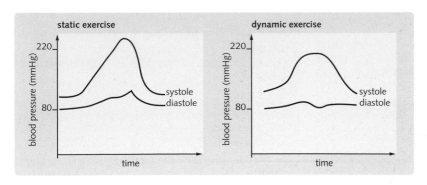

Fig. 4.11 Blood pressure during static and dynamic exercise. Diastolic pressure rises in static exercise, but it remains relatively constant in dynamic exercise. The cardiac work is greater for equivalent static than for dynamic exercise.

exercise pressor response, which is mediated by receptors in the muscle.

Initiation of the response to exercise

The exact causes of the changes in autonomic activity during exercise are not known. Two hypotheses are prevalent:

- The central command hypothesis. This postulates that as the cerebral cortex initiates contraction of muscle, it also instructs the autonomic nerves of the brainstem to increase heart rate. Baroreflex resetting to a higher value may also be linked to this theory.
- The peripheral reflex hypothesis. The nerve receptors in working muscle are excited by the presence of chemical stimulants, and they cause a reflex sympathetic response, increasing cardiac output and pressure.

It is likely that the central command hypothesis produces the initial tachycardia and vagal suppression. The peripheral reflex hypothesis probably accounts for the slower increase in cardiac output and peripheral vasoconstriction.

Cardiovascular response to training

This is most important in the long-distance or endurance athlete. Training causes improvement in oxygen transport rate and changes in cardiac structure and function. Causes of improved oxygen delivery and extraction are:

- New capillaries formed in skeletal muscle.
- More muscle mitochondria closer to capillaries.
- Increased muscle myoglobin concentration.

Changes in cardiac structure and function are:

- Thicker ventricular wall.
- Increased myocardial vascularity.
- Increased ventricular cavity size.

Stroke volume is much higher because of the cardiac changes. Most athletes have a resting bradycardia, but because of the increased stroke volume the resting cardiac output is the same.

In exercise, the athlete's maximum heart rate is the same as that for an untrained subject, but because the athlete starts at a lower value, a much greater change can be achieved. This, coupled with the increased stroke volume, means that the athlete can increase cardiac output up to as much as 35 L/min.

Diving reflex

The diving reflex occurs when cold water touches the facial receptors of the trigeminal nerve. The body is expecting a dive into water and a period of submersion. The limited oxygen must be preferentially diverted to the heart and brain. There are three reflexes involved:

- Apnoea – arterial chemoreceptors are triggered as asphyxia develops.
- Bradycardia – caused by intense vagal inhibition of the pacemaker.
- Peripheral vasoconstriction – occurs in the splanchnic, renal and skeletal muscle vascular beds. The strong, sympathetically mediated vasoconstriction overwhelms any metabolic dilatation that may occur in active muscle.

In marine mammals, the diving reflex is much stronger and, coupled with their larger store of oxygen and myoglobin, this enables them to survive submerged for longer periods.

Syncope

Syncope (see p. 138) is a sudden, transient loss of consciousness as a result of impaired cerebral perfusion. It is caused by a drop in cerebral blood flow to less than half its normal value.

It may be initiated by a pathophysiological cause (e.g. orthostasis or severe hypovolaemia) or by psychological stress (e.g. fear, pain, or horror). In psychogenic fainting, there is often a pre-faint period of tachycardia, cutaneous vasoconstriction, hyperventilation, and sweating. A vasovagal episode (frequently a faint) proceeds as follows:

1. A sudden increase in vagal inhibition leads to bradycardia.
2. Peripheral vasodilatation results due to decreased sympathetic drive.
3. This causes a fall in blood pressure, reducing cerebral blood flow.
4. If it occurs at all, loss of consciousness results within seconds.

Fits, faints and funny turns are very common presentations of cardiovascular disease. It is important to consider a number of pathologies in the nervous, cardiovascular and respiratory systems before reaching the diagnosis of a psychological cause. A thorough history and an open mind will help prevent you from making mistakes!

The cause of the sudden changes is unknown. In psychogenic fainting, it could be a primitive 'playing dead' response. In hypovolaemic fainting, it could be triggered by mechanoreceptors in the near-empty left ventricle.

The person who has fainted ends up in the supine position. This raises the intrathoracic blood volume and the filling pressure. Coupled with the baroreflex, this then increases cardiac output and arterial pressure. Consciousness is restored in under 2 minutes.

The cardiovascular system in disease – diseases of the heart

5

Objectives

You should be able to:

- Describe the various presentations of ischaemic heart disease.
- Recall the risk factors for ischaemic heart disease, and link these to treatment principles.
- Understand in detail the pathology and treatment of myocardial infarction.
- Understand the pathology, presentation, clinical features and treatment of heart failure.
- Understand the origin and character of the most common arrhythmias.
- Describe the common causes of valvular lesions.
- Understand the diseases which commonly affect the myocardium
- Understand the diseases which commonly affect the pericardium.
- Describe and draw the common congenital defects affecting the heart and great vessels.
- Be aware of the neoplastic conditions which may arise in the heart.

ISCHAEMIC HEART DISEASE

Myocardial ischaemia occurs when the blood supply to the myocardium is insufficient for its needs. This can be due to:

- An impaired blood supply to the myocardium.
- An increased demand by the myocardium.

Ischaemia can also occur because of reduced oxygen transport (e.g. in shock, severe anaemia, lung disease and congenital heart disease) and may contribute significantly to damage if it occurs with the above.

Ischaemic heart disease (also called coronary heart disease) is the leading cause of death in the Western world (30% of male and 23% of female deaths). It is mainly caused by atherosclerosis of the coronary arteries, and more commonly affects the left ventricle because of its larger size and demand (see p. 91). The main clinical syndromes are either chronic or acute. Risk factors for ischaemic heart disease are summarized in Fig. 5.1.

The aetiology of ischaemic heart disease is usually a result of complications of atherosclerotic plaques in the coronary arteries, which can be:

- Progressive atherosclerosis leading to stenosis.
- Thrombus formation on a plaque caused by superficial ulceration.
- Plaque fissuring, leading to thrombus formation in the lumen or haemorrhage into the plaque.

Knowledge of the risk factors for ischaemic heart disease is absolutely essential, both for examinations and clinical practice. Modification of these risk factors is the mainstay of both primary and secondary prevention.

Vasospasm may precipitate these changes or reduce coronary blood flow on its own (e.g. in Prinzmetal's angina). Ischaemia can also result from:

- Narrowing of the coronary ostia in syphilis or atherosclerosis.
- Emboli as a result of infective endocarditis, or other causes such as thromboembolism.

constitutional	modifiable
sex (male)	smoking
age	diabetes
family history	hypertension
previous personal history	hypercholesterolaemia
	pro-thrombotic state
	excessive alcohol
	physical inactivity and obesity
	stress

Fig. 5.1 Constitutional and modifiable risk factors for ischaemic heart disease.

- Arteritides (e.g. polyarteritis nodosa, Kawasaki's syndrome).
- Shock caused by haemorrhage.
- Severe aortic valvular disease.
- Severe anaemia.

Acute ischaemic heart disease

Unstable angina (or crescendo angina) is a sudden onset of angina, caused by the fissuring of atherosclerotic plaques. Myocardial infarction occurs when a region of the myocardium fails to be perfused with blood and becomes necrotic. This may be subendocardial (a superficial injury), or transmural (full thickness), see p. 80.

Sudden cardiac death is usually caused by ventricular fibrillation secondary to an acute myocardial infarction.

Chronic ischaemic heart disease

Chronic ischaemic heart disease occurs predominantly in elderly persons with severe atherosclerosis of many coronary vessels. Patients may progressively develop congestive cardiac failure. Atrophy of the myocytes and diffuse fibrosis can be seen microscopically. Death may be caused by:

- Cardiac failure.
- Acute myocardial infarction.
- Arrhythmia.

Angina pectoris

Angina pectoris literally means 'a choking sensation in the chest'. It is an episodic pain that usually occurs in the centre of the chest, often radiating to the neck and left arm and frequently induced by exercise. It is commonly classified as:

- Angina of effort (classic angina) – occurs after exertion, excitation or emotion and is caused by an insufficient oxygen supply to meet an increased demand. Classically, the pain subsides with rest. It may be stable (gradual stenosis by a progressive plaque build-up) or unstable (sudden plaque fissuring producing thrombosis).
- Vasospastic (Prinzmetal's) angina – caused by transient spasm of the coronary artery obstructing blood flow.

Angina occurs because myocardial oxygen requirement is greater than its supply. This leads to a build-up in local metabolites causing pain.

Medical treatment of angina

Treatment strategies for angina involve increasing oxygen supply to the ischaemic zone and decreasing oxygen demand of the myocardium. Increasing oxygen supply to the ischaemic zone can be achieved by dilating the coronary arteries or decreasing heart rate:

- Coronary arteries predominantly supply blood during diastole. With a slower heart rate there is less cardiac work, less demand for blood supply yet a prolonged period of diastole, giving more time for perfusion of the myocardium.
- Dilating coronary arteries (e.g. with Ca^{2+} antagonists) are very useful in angina where there is incomplete or irregular dilatation.

Decreasing the oxygen demand of the myocardium can be achieved by two methods:

- Directly decreasing force and heart rate (β-blockers, Ca^{2+} antagonists).
- Decreasing the pressure necessary to overcome systemic vascular resistance with vasodilators and venodilators (nitrates, nicorandil, Ca^{2+} antagonists; reduce afterload).

Active control of risk factors is also a key component of long-term management, and this should not be neglected (e.g. smoking cessation, regular exercise, and dietary control). The following are commonly used anti-anginals.

Organic nitrates

Organic nitrates, e.g. glyceryl trinitrate (GTN), act by relaxing vascular smooth muscle by producing NO in smooth muscle, which increases cyclic guanosine monophosphate (cGMP) and brings about dilatation. The greatest effect is on venous capacitance vessels, increasing venous pooling and, therefore, reducing heart size, and myocardial oxygen demand.

Organic nitrates are used in both angina of effort and vasospastic angina:

- Angina of effort. By Starling's law, decreased venous return results in decreased cardiac output and, therefore, oxygen demand.
- Vasospastic angina. Nitrates have a direct dilatory effect on the coronary arteries, reducing spasm.

GTN is subject to first-pass metabolism, and it is, therefore, taken sublingually. The effect lasts for approximately 30 min. It is used to stop or prevent an angina attack. Longer acting nitrates include isosorbide mononitrate and isosorbide dinitrate. Side effects are:

- Postural or systemic hypotension.
- Reflex tachycardia.
- Headache and facial flushing.
- Tolerance (may develop over 2–3 days of continuous use).

Calcium channel blockers (e.g. amlodipine, nifedipine, verapamil, diltiazem)

These drugs block Ca^{2+} channels, decreasing contraction of smooth and cardiac muscle. In addition, verapamil and diltiazem will both decrease heart rate. They mainly cause vasodilatation, and they are used in both angina of effort and vasospastic angina:

- Angina of effort. Calcium channel blockers decrease total peripheral resistance, lessening the demand on the heart.
- Vasospastic angina. These drugs cause relaxation of spasm.

Side effects of calcium channel blockers are:

- Headache and facial flushing.
- Constipation.
- Reflex tachycardia.
- Oedema.

Due to their negative chronotropic effects, caution should be exercised when using verapamil and diltiazem in combination with β-blockers, as profound bradycardia may result. Nifedipine, however, may be beneficially combined with β-blockers to minimize reflex tachycardia.

Potassium channel agonists

Potassium channel agonists (e.g. nicorandil) act by opening ATP-dependent K^+ channels in vascular smooth muscle, making depolarization more difficult to achieve and leading to vasodilatation and venodilation. This reduces heart size, and myocardial oxygen demand.

Potassium channel agonists are an alternative to nitrates when tolerance occurs and if β-blockers and Ca^{2+} antagonists are contraindicated. Nicorandil has some nitrate effects. Other side effects include:

- Headache and facial flushing.
- Postural hypotension.
- Weakness.

Beta-blockers

These drugs block sympathetic stimulation of the heart, leading to:

- Decreased force and, therefore, decreased oxygen demand.
- Decreased rate and, therefore, decreased oxygen demand and also increased time for oxygen supply (prolonged diastole).

They are used in angina of effort, but not in vasospastic angina as they have no dilatory effect. They should not be used to treat patients with asthma or bradyarrhythmias, and should be used cautiously in patients with peripheral arterial disease.

Many drugs of the same class have similar suffixes to their names. For example, most β-blockers end in '-ol' (e.g. propranolol, atenolol, metoprolol). This is useful when identifying the class of an unfamiliar drug.

Surgical treatment of angina

These should be considered when:

- There is a lesion that can be treated by an appropriate technique.
- General measures and medical treatment have failed to relieve the symptoms.

- The benefits of coronary revascularization outweigh the risk of the procedure.

Percutaneous coronary intervention

Percutaneous transluminal coronary angioplasty (PTCA) uses information gained from a coronary angiogram, which shows the state of the coronary vasculature. It is usually used for the treatment of isolated, proximal, non-calcified atheromatous plaques, but it can be used for multiple lesions and it can be repeated.

The method involves the use of a balloon, usually inserted via the femoral artery, which is inflated in the stenosed artery to cause dilation. The balloon is inserted past the obstruction in the artery using x-ray fluoroscopy and then inflated with a contrast material. Multiple inflations of the balloon compress and crack the atheroma, reducing the obstruction.

New interventions are being developed constantly, and include the use of atherectomy devices (for removal of plaque) and ablative techniques.

Complications include:

- Acute coronary occlusion.
- Re-stenosis (occurs in 30% in first 6 months).

Outcome can be improved using a device called a stent – a metallic 'scaffold' – that is introduced around the balloon catheter. Inflation of the balloon fixes the stent in position, reducing the risk of re-stenosis. Drug-eluting stents are now becoming more common; an antiproliferative agent is impregnated into a polymer which coats the stent, promoting longevity.

Coronary artery bypass graft (CABG)

For left anterior descending (LAD) artery lesions, the left internal mammary artery is detached distally and anastomosed distal to the coronary artery stenosis. A conduit is used to bypass obstructions in other vessels, and may be an artery (e.g. right internal mammary or radial) or vein (usually the long saphenous from the leg). It is usually attached from the aorta to the artery distal to the obstruction. Multiple obstructions can by dealt with by these methods. Considerable improvement is achieved from the surgery in about 90% of cases (Fig. 5.2).

Complications include:

- Mortality (about 1%).
- Slow occlusion of the grafts.

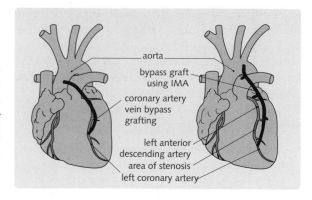

Fig. 5.2 Coronary artery bypass graft using a leg vein and left internal mammary artery (IMA). (Redrawn with permission from Thelan I A, et al. Critical care nursing: diagnosis and management, 2nd edn. London: Mosby, 1994.)

Myocardial infarction

Myocardial infarction is classified as:

- Subendocardial myocardial infarction – affecting the innermost region of the myocardium.
- Transmural myocardial infarction – affecting the full thickness of one segment of the myocardium.

Myocardial infarction occurs when an area of myocardium dies (i.e. undergoes necrosis). It is caused by a reduction or blockage in the coronary blood supply, and it is usually precipitated by thrombosis (or rarely haemorrhage) in an atherosclerotic area of a coronary artery. There are many complications including arrhythmias, heart failure, and even sudden death.

A subendocardial infarction affects the subendocardial layer of the myocardium, whereas a transmural infarction affects the full thickness of the myocardium. An infarct usually occurs as the result of occlusion of a major coronary artery, causing ischaemia to a specific region of the heart. This may be caused by:

- An acute plaque change (ulceration, fissuring or haemorrhage) leading to thrombosis.
- Platelet aggregation.
- Hypotension (rarely).
- Vasospasm (rarely).

Complete occlusion of a vessel may not cause infarction as collaterals may have developed, aiding perfusion.

Nearly all infarcts affect the left ventricle; 15% involve both ventricles, and 3% involve just the right ventricle. The arteries commonly infarcted are:

- Left anterior descending artery (50%) – affecting the left ventricular anterior wall and interventricular septum.
- Right coronary artery (30%) – affecting the left ventricular inferior and posterior walls and right ventricle.
- Left circumflex artery (20%) – affecting the left ventricular lateral wall.

From the onset of ischaemia, it takes only 20–40 minutes until irreversible injury starts to occur. Reperfusion (the return of flow) caused by thrombolysis (spontaneous, drug or surgically induced) can lessen the extent of damage. Reperfused myocytes may not function to the same level for a few days. A characteristic series of events occurs (Fig. 5.3).

Sudden death occurs in 25% of patients, usually as a result of an arrhythmia; 90% of survivors develop acute or chronic complications. Acute complications include:

- Arrhythmias.
- Heart failure.
- Cardiogenic shock.
- Ventricular rupture.
- Papillary muscle infarction, leading to mitral valve incompetence.
- Mural thrombosis, leading to pulmonary or peripheral thromboembolism.
- Pericarditis.

Chronic complications include:

- Ventricular aneurysm and thrombosis.
- Recurrent infarction.
- Arrhythmias.
- Chronic heart failure.
- Dressler's syndrome (autoimmune inflammatory pericarditis and effusions).

Mortality is 35% in the first year, and 10% every year thereafter.

The acute admission with ischaemic heart disease is very common. Any patient with cardiac chest pain should be treated as if they have an acute coronary syndrome. The initial management, as with any acute patient, is – Airway, Breathing, Circulation. The patient should have a 12-lead ECG. First line treatment is MONA (morphine, oxygen, nitrates, aspirin). After this clopidogrel, thrombolytic therapy and primary coronary intervention should be considered.

Treatment

The treatment of myocardial infarction centres around the modification of risk factors for ischaemic heart disease (see p. 78), and the treatment of angina (see p. 79). There are however some additional therapies which may be utilized.

Fibrinolytic drugs

Thrombolytic (fibrinolytic) therapy is used to break down the thrombi that cause a myocardial infarction. If given within 3 hours, it probably allows reperfusion in about half of the affected arteries.

Thrombolytics include:

- (Recombinant) tissue plasminogen activator (rTPA), e.g. tenecteplase, reteplase. This group of drugs is increasingly being used for all

Events occurring after myocardial infarction		
Time after myocardial infarction	Macroscopic events	Microscopic events
6–12 h	Normal	Oedema
12–18 h	Normal	Neutrophils appear
18–24 h	Pale or cyanotic	Myocyte necrosis
1–3 days	Hyperaemic border	Inflammation
3–7 days	Yellow, sharply defined lesion that softens	Dead cells disintegrate and are mopped up by macrophages
7–10 days	Haemorrhagic edge	Granulation tissue replaces dead tissue
12 days	Scar formation	Dense fibrous tissue

Fig. 5.3 Time line of events occurring after infarction.

infarcts meeting thrombolytic criteria as a result of the GUSTO trials (a series of global studies of cardiovascular disease treatments), which showed them to be more efficacious than streptokinase. These drugs must be given with heparin.

- Streptokinase – binds and activates plasminogen to form plasmin, causing fibrinolysis. Plasmin also lyses fibrinogen and prothrombin (anticoagulant effect). Streptokinase cannot be used repeatedly as antibodies are generated which may induce anaphylaxis on subsequent exposure.

There are strict criteria for the administration of thrombolytic agents, as outlined in Fig. 5.4. Side effects of these agents include:

- Nausea and vomiting.
- Bleeding (may result in strokes).

Primary percutaneous coronary intervention

Some centres now use primary 'rescue' angioplasty (see above) to relieve the obstruction which resulted in infarction. This may be used as a first-line intervention, or more commonly following failed thrombolytic therapy.

Non-steroidal anti-inflammatory drugs (NSAIDs)

Aspirin is an NSAID that irreversibly inhibits the cyclo-oxygenase (COX) enzyme. It has been shown to be beneficial in an acute myocardial infarction (with streptokinase) and in preventing myocardial infarction and stroke.

Aspirin's beneficial effects in thromboembolic disease are thought to be caused by decreased synthesis of thromboxane A_2 (Tx-A_2) by platelets. Tx-A_2 is a strong inducer of platelet aggregation. Its action is antagonized by prostacyclin (PGI_2) from endothelial cells. PGI_2 synthesis is also blocked by aspirin, but the endothelial cell is able to produce more COX enzyme (this cannot occur in platelets as they have no nucleus). The overall action, therefore, is to favour non-aggregation of platelets. Side effects include:

- Bronchospasm.
- Gastrointestinal haemorrhage.

Clopidogrel is increasingly being used as an adjunct or alternative to aspirin. The mechanism of action of clopidogrel is irreversible blockade of the adenosine diphosphate (ADP) receptor on platelet cell membranes. This receptor is named P2Y12 and is important in platelet aggregation. The blockade of this receptor inhibits platelet aggregation by blocking activation of the glycoprotein IIb/IIIa pathway. Clopidogrel is used in the treatment of both ST elevation and non-ST elevation myocardial infarction (see p. 80), and also in secondary prevention of ischaemic heart disease.

Sudden cardiac death

Sudden cardiac death is unexpected death from a cardiac cause within 1 hour of onset of symptoms. There is usually plaque disruption, but ultimately death is caused by a fatal arrhythmia (asystole or ventricular fibrillation) due to scarring of the conduction system, acute ischaemic injury, or electrolyte imbalance.

HEART FAILURE

Definition

Heart failure (cardiac failure) is said to have occurred when the heart is no longer able to maintain sufficient tissue perfusion for normal cellular metabolism.

Conditions

Conditions that lead to heart failure can be divided into:

- Those that damage cardiac muscle (e.g. ischaemic heart disease, cardiomyopathies).
- Those that demand extra work of the heart (e.g. systemic hypertension, valvular heart disease).

Remember, 'heart failure' is NOT a diagnosis. It is always necessary to identify the underlying pathology responsible, so that a targeted treatment regime can be employed.

Symptoms and signs

Symptoms and signs of heart failure are dependent on the ventricle which is primarily affected. The above mentioned conditions affect the left ventricle,

indications	absolute contraindications	relative contraindications (discuss with cardiologist)
• chest pain for less than 12 hours and 1 of: A) ST elevation more than 1 mm in 2 adjacent limb leads B) ST elevation more than 2 mm in 2 adjacent chest leads C) new onset left bundle branch block (LBBB) D) ST depression in V1–V4 with R wave in V1–V2 (suspected posterior infarct)	• active bleeding • known bleeding disorder • major surgery or trauma within last 4 weeks • recent non-compressible vascular puncture • haemorrhagic CVA in previous year • CVA of unknown type within last 6 weeks • pregnancy	• potential serious bleeding • prolonged CPR (>5 min) • severe liver disease • severe diabetic retinopathy • uncontrolled hypertension • ongoing oral anticoagulation • active peptic ulcer

Fig. 5.4 Indications and contraindications for thrombolytic therapy.

resulting in a build-up of fluid into the pulmonary circulation and subsequent pulmonary oedema. Right ventricular failure (most commonly caused by left ventricular failure) results in a build-up of fluid into the systemic circulation and subsequent oedema. Together, this picture is referred to as congestive cardiac failure, the signs and symptoms of which include:

- Muscle fatigue.
- Reduced exercise tolerance.
- Tachycardia.
- Dyspnoea, possibly caused by increased fluid in the lungs.
- Orthopnoea (shortness of breath while lying flat).
- Paroxysmal nocturnal dyspnoea (sudden shortness of breath while sleeping).
- Haemoptysis caused by increased venous pressure, leading to alveolar haemorrhage.
- Elevated jugular venous pressure (due to venous congestion).
- Hepatomegaly (due to venous congestion).
- Oedema (due to venous congestion).
- Proteinuria (due to prerenal renal failure).

Compensatory mechanisms

There is a decrease in contractility of the affected heart muscle in chronic heart failure from left ventricular systolic dysfunction. This shifts the Starling curve to the right and reduces the force of contraction for a given filling pressure (Fig. 5.5). The body attempts to compensate by increasing filling pressure (Fig. 5.6).

This is achieved by:

- Catecholamine release causing increased sympathetic nerve activity, increasing heart rate and force.
- Peripheral vasoconstriction/venoconstriction, which will increase filling pressure but also total peripheral resistance (this increases the demand on the heart).
- Renal retention of Na^+ and water to increase blood volume and filling pressure, also causing oedema.

These responses only confer a limited improvement. Increased cardiac filling initially increases cardiac output through Starling's law, but prolonged excessive cardiac filling causes persisting dilatation. This leads to ineffective contraction and causes the heart to enlarge and eventually fail. According to Laplace's law, dilatation of the heart requires the myocytes to increase the tension in the wall to sustain the same pressure (see p. 17). This increases oxygen demand and predisposes the myocardium to ischaemia. Dilatation may also ultimately lead to valvular incompetence (see p. 90). A key aim for treatment is, therefore, to reduce the load on the failing heart, e.g. by venodilation, although this carries a risk of precipitating cardiogenic shock.

Increased catecholamine release (i.e. increased sympathetic drive) results in increased adrenaline and noradrenaline secretion to increase the force and rate of contraction. As the condition worsens, there is an eventual downregulation of β-adrenoceptors reducing this effect.

Treatment of heart failure

Heart failure can present as an acute emergency (pulmonary oedema) or a chronic condition (pedal oedema). Pulmonary oedema occurs as the result of left-sided heart failure, whereas pedal oedema occurs as the result of right-sided heart failure. Treatment should be focussed on maintaining longevity and improving quality of life, i.e. removing excess fluid and addressing cardiovascular risk factors.

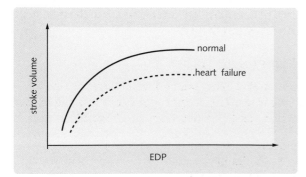

Fig. 5.5 The Starling curve in heart failure. Reduced contractility reduces stroke volume for a given filling pressure (EDP, end-diastolic pressure).

Angiotensin-converting enzyme inhibitors

ACE inhibitors (e.g. enalapril, lisinopril, and captopril):

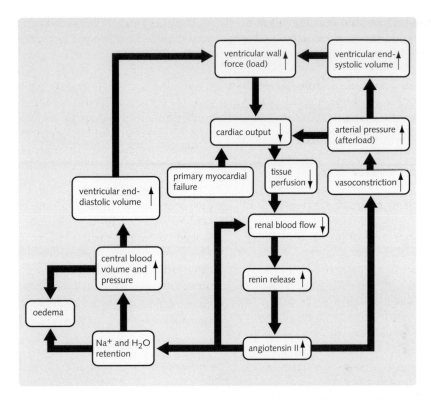

Fig. 5.6 The series of changes in heart failure is initiated by myocardial changes, which impair the efficiency of the heart. Causes include infarction, cardiomyopathy, and chronic hypertension. In the normal heart, an increased end-diastolic or systolic volume leads to greater cardiac output by Starling's law, but in a heart with impaired contractility there is little further reserve. Dilatation of the ventricles further impairs the efficiency of the heart by Laplace's law, requiring greater effort to maintain output.

Compensatory changes include sympathetic activation to increase contractility and to raise blood pressure, in order to maintain tissue perfusion, but chronic stimulation leads to an impaired adrenergic response. The renin–angiotensin system is also activated, leading to fluid retention and raised blood pressure.

Attempts to raise the systemic blood pressure place further load on an already weakened heart, creating a destructive cycle. Therapy is aimed at controlling these compensatory mechanisms to unload the heart and prevent excessive dilatation.

- Block production of angiotensin II and, therefore, aldosterone.
- Prevent the breakdown of bradykinin.
- Prolong life in heart failure.

ACE inhibitors produce vasodilatation/venodilatation, thereby decreasing afterload and subsequent oedema (ACE inhibitors are also used in hypertension, see p. 110).

Beta-blockers

The sympatholytic effects of β-blockers (see p. 79) have been shown to be beneficial in the long-term management of heart failure. Their action slows the heart, thereby increasing filling time while allowing β-receptor sensitivity to recover. They should be used with caution however, and not in the treatment of acute heart failure.

Diuretics

Diuretics increase salt and water excretion, therefore decreasing circulatory volume. This decreases preload and oedema. They are classified as:

- Thiazides.
- Loop diuretics.
- Potassium-sparing diuretics.

Thiazides are used in mild cardiac failure and hypertension (see p. 110), whereas loop diuretics are reserved for moderate and severe heart failure. Potassium-sparing diuretics are sometimes used in conjunction with other diuretics to prevent hypokalaemia.

Diuretics are often used in combination with an ACE inhibitor.

Thiazides

Thiazides (e.g. chlorothiazide, bendroflumethiazide, metolazone) prevent Na^+ and Cl^- reabsorption in the distal tubule. Side effects are:

- Hypokalaemia.
- Hyperuricaemia.
- Hypercholesterolaemia.
- Hyperglycaemia.

Loop diuretics

Loop diuretics (e.g. frusemide and bumetanide) inhibit NaCl reabsorption in the loop of Henle. They cause more potent diuresis than other diuretics, and they can be used in patients with reduced renal function. Side effects are:

- Those of thiazides.
- Deafness at high doses.

Potassium-sparing diuretics

Potassium-sparing diuretics (e.g. spironolactone and amiloride) antagonize the effect of aldosterone, or block Na^+ channels, at the distal tubule. This prevents Na^+ reabsorption and K^+ excretion. Spironolactone has been shown to prolong life in heart failure. The main side effect is hyperkalaemia, a major risk when combined with ACE inhibitors.

Inotropic drugs

Inotropic drugs increase the contractility of the myocardium. Their principal role should be restricted to the management of acute heart failure, as they are associated with increased mortality with long-term use.

They can be classified as:

- Cardiac glycosides.
- β_1-sympathomimetics.
- Phosphodiesterase inhibitors.

Cardiac glycosides

Cardiac glycosides (e.g. digoxin and ouabain) inhibit the Na^+/K^+ pump, which leads to a rise in intracellular Ca^{2+}. This:

- Increases the force of contraction.
- Reduces the heart's oxygen consumption.

They also have a central effect to increase vagal activity, which slows the heart rate.

The side effects of cardiac glycosides are:

- Anorexia.
- Nausea and vomiting.
- Diarrhoea.
- Confusion.
- Arrhythmia in toxic doses.

Cardiac glycosides are contraindicated in hypokalaemia because of potentiation of their action, and they should be combined with thiazides and loop diuretics with caution.

β_1-Sympathomimetics

The β_1-sympathomimetics dobutamine and dopamine increase the force of contraction. Dopamine also increases renal blood flow in low doses. Side effects are tachycardia and hypertension in overdose.

Phosphodiesterase inhibitors (milrinone)

Milrinone (caffeine) inhibits phosphodiesterase, which is the enzyme that breaks down cyclic adenosine monophosphate (cAMP) into 5'-AMP. Inhibition causes a rise in intracellular cAMP and, therefore, Ca^{2+}. This means there is an increase in contractility. Milrinone is also a vasodilator. It is used in severe heart failure that is unresponsive to other therapy.

Non-drug treatment of heart failure

Cardiac resynchronization therapy (CRT)

Patients with heart failure often have left bundle branch block. As the conduction system in these individuals is abnormal, the pathway of repolarization is also abnormal and the heart does not contract uniformly (there is some dys-synchrony in the ventricular contraction). New pacemakers have been developed that stimulate both the right and the left ventricle simultaneously, with the obvious benefit of resynchronizing the depolarization of the left and right ventricles. This increases cardiac output and does appear to be of benefit in patients with heart failure and broad QRS complexes.

Implantable cardiac defibrillators (ICDs)

Patients with heart failure are prone to malignant arrhythmias. ICDs can be implanted in a similar way to pacemaker devices to deliver a small electrical impulse when an arrhythmia arises, preventing sudden cardiac death.

Heart transplantation

Many procedures are still in the experimental phase, including the fitting of ventricular assist devices to encourage ventricular systolic function. The mainstay of surgical treatment of heart failure however is still heart transplantation.

Heart transplantation has become the treatment of choice for severe, intractable heart failure in younger patients. Life expectancy would be about 6 months without radical intervention. The procedure requires the use of ciclosporin for immunosuppression. With good patient selection, the prognosis is good, with one-year survival rates of 80% and 5-year survival of 70%. The quality of life of the majority of patients is dramatically improved.

ARRHYTHMIA

Definitions and classification

An arrhythmia is any deviation from the heart's normal sinus rhythm. Descriptions of arrhythmias are outlined below. Arrhythmias are usually classified clinically as supraventricular or ventricular.

- Supraventricular – originating in the atrium or atrioventricular node.
- Ventricular – originating in the ventricle.

Altered sinus rhythms

Sinus tachycardia and sinus bradycardia are produced by autonomic nervous activity. It usually takes several beats to produce a new steady state.

Tachycardia (>100 beats/min in adults) usually results from:

- Exercise.
- Emotion.
- Fever.

Sinus tachycardia will show normal P waves, with a stable P–R interval within normal limits.

Bradycardia (<60 beats/min) commonly occurs in:

- Athletes.
- Patients with raised intracranial pressure.

Sinus arrhythmia generally manifests in the young as a change in rhythm with respiration. The heart rate increases with inspiration and decreases with expiration.

Extrasystole (ectopic beats)

Extrasystole occurs when an abnormal beat is generated in an area of myocardium before the next sinus beat. The impulse that is generated goes on to contract the ventricle. Atrial extrasystole (narrow and regular) or ventricular extrasystole (broad and irregular) may occur, depending upon the area of origin. Usually, there is a gap before the next normal sinus beat; this is termed the compensatory phase (see p. 27)

Wolff–Parkinson–White syndrome

In Wolff–Parkinson–White syndrome there is an extra conduction pathway (the bundle of Kent) between the atria and ventricles. This results in rapid conduction, which can lead to tachycardia or atrial fibrillation.

Atrial arrhythmias

Supraventricular tachycardia and atrial flutter

Atrial tachycardia and atrial flutter are caused by an abnormal focus in the atrium or an abnormal conduction pathway causing re-entry that results in atrial contraction at a rapid rate. It may also be caused by ectopic or junctional beats that may arise from the myocardium surrounding the atrioventricular node, or the tissue forming the 'junctional area' which connects the atrioventricular node to the ventricular conduction system. Ectopic beats or abnormal conduction (e.g. Wolff–Parkinson–White, ischaemia) within this area may produce an atrioventricular re-entry tachycardia. P waves may be inverted on an ECG, but they may still cause atrial or ventricular contraction.

In atrial flutter the rate is usually around 300 beats/min but not all atrial impulses are conducted to the ventricle. Often, the ratio of atrial to ventricular beats is 2 : 1 or 3 : 1 (i.e. a variable atrioventricular heart block, see below).

Supraventricular tachycardia is characterized by a heart rate usually between 140 and 220 beats/min, with narrow QRS complexes.

Atrial fibrillation

There is no coordinated atrial activity in atrial fibrillation. A rippling effect of the muscle occurs, which does not contribute to ventricular filling. Ventricular activity is affected, producing a characteristic 'irregularly irregular' pulse in rate and volume. It is commonly caused by mitral valve disease, ischaemic heart disease, thyrotoxicosis, hypertension and alcohol.

> Arrhythmias are very common and often go unnoticed by the patient. The treatment of atrial fibrillation has three domains. Firstly, it is possible to cardiovert the patient back to sinus rhythm, either chemically or electrically. Secondly, it is important to control the rate of the arrhythmia in order to allow adequate ventricular filling. Thirdly, due to the increased risk of thromboembolism, a longstanding arrhythmia is an indication for anticoagulation.

Heart block (atrioventricular block)

This is an interruption of the normal conduction through the atrioventricular conduction tissue. It may be classified as first-, second-, or third-degree block.

First-degree heart block

In first-degree heart block, all atrial impulses reach the ventricle, but conduction through the atrioventricular tissue takes longer than normal (P–R interval on an electrocardiogram is >0.2 s).

Second-degree heart block

In second-degree heart block, some atrial impulses fail to reach the ventricles, but others do (not all P waves are followed by QRS complexes).

Mobitz type 1 (Wenckebach) heart block
In Wenckebach heart block, the degree of block increases over a few beats (P–R interval increases over three or four beats, followed by an isolated P wave). This is analogous to a 'lazy' node which can still function.

Mobitz type 2 heart block
This is characterized by an unexpected non-conducted atrial impulse. Thus, the P–R and R–R intervals between conducted beats are constant. This is analogous to a fracture in the His–Purkinje system

which is about to become completely severed. This frequently progresses to complete heart block and is associated with a progression to sudden cardiac death.

Third-degree (complete) heart block

In third-degree heart block, the atria and ventricles beat independently of each other. The ventricular rate is usually about 20–40 beats/min (P waves and QRS complexes have no fixed relationship).

Ventricular arrhythmias

Ventricular arrhythmias commonly present as a cardiac arrest (see p. 139).

Ventricular tachycardia

Ventricular tachycardia occurs when impulses originate from an ectopic focus within the ventricles. It is characterized by broad QRS complexes (i.e. duration >100 ms) on an ECG at a rate of >120 beats/min. This arrhythmia is not usually associated with an effective cardiac output.

Ventricular fibrillation

Ventricular fibrillation is an irregular uncoordinated rippling contraction of the ventricle. There is no effective cardiac output, leading to rapid loss of consciousness. Death results unless effective treatment is initiated immediately.

Mechanism of arrhythmia

Arrhythmias are caused by a combination of abnormal impulse generation (either an abnormal sinus rhythm or an ectopic pacemaker), delayed depolarization after an action potential (which can result in a second contraction), and re-entry. A more detailed account of arrhythmia is given in Chapter 9.

Anti-arrhythmic drugs

The aims of drug treatment are:

- To decrease cell excitability.
- To increase the refractory period.
- To slow conduction or block conduction if already slow.

The Vaughan-Williams classification system is used for anti-arrhythmic drugs; it is based on their actions.

Class I: sodium channel blockers

These drugs can be subdivided into class IA (e.g. quinidine, procainamide, disopyramide), class IB (e.g. lignocaine, mexiletine, tocainide), and class IC (e.g. flecainide). They block sodium channels during the open (classes IA and IC) or refractory (class IB) state. They are all 'use-dependent' blockers, only affecting active channels.

Class IA: quinidine, procainamide, disopyramide

Class IA drugs prolong the action potential by:

- Increasing the threshold for spontaneous depolarization.
- Slowing the fast upstroke.
- Prolonging the refractory period.

These drugs are used for supraventricular and ventricular arrhythmias. Side effects include:

- Nausea and vomiting.
- Anticholinergic effects – dry mouth, blurred vision, and urinary retention.
- Hypotension (disopyramide).
- Precipitation of systemic lupus erythematosus (procainamide).

Class IB: lignocaine (lidocaine), mexiletine, tocainide

Class IB drugs bind preferentially to refractory Na^+ channels, and so they act preferentially on ischaemic myocardium. They shorten the action potential by:

- Slowing the fast upstroke.
- Increasing the refractory period.

They are used for ventricular arrhythmias, especially after a myocardial infarction. Side effects include:

- Convulsions.
- Nausea and vomiting.

Class IC: flecainide, propafenone

Class IC drugs have little effect on action potential, but they slow upstroke and conduction speed; there is little change in refractory period. They are used in supraventricular and ventricular arrhythmias. Side effects include:

- Further arrhythmias.
- Dizziness.

Class II: β-adrenergic blockers

Class II drugs (e.g. propranolol and atenolol) block the increase in pacemaker activity that is produced by sympathetic stimulation of β-adrenoceptors. They also slow conduction.

Beta-blockers may be used for ectopic beats, atrial fibrillation and atrial tachycardia. They are indicated when circulating catecholamines are too high (e.g. after a myocardial infarction and thyrotoxicosis). Side effects are:

- Tiredness.
- Provoke asthma.

Some drugs (such as sotalol and bretylium) have both class II and III actions.

Class III: potassium channel blockers

Class III drugs (e.g. amiodarone) block K^+ channels, slowing repolarization leading to a prolonged action potential and refractory period.

Class III drugs are used in supraventricular and ventricular arrhythmias. Side effects of amiodarone are important and common. They include:

- Photosensitivity (an increased tendency to sunburn).
- Blue/grey discolouration of the skin.
- Liver toxicity.
- Thyroid disorders.
- Neuropathy.
- Pulmonary alveolitis.

Amiodarone also has class IA and II effects.

Class IV: calcium channel blockers

Class IV drugs (e.g. verapamil) block Ca^{2+} channels, thereby decreasing spontaneous activity and conduction at sinoatrial and atrioventricular nodes.

Class IV drugs are used for supraventricular arrhythmias only. Side effects of verapamil include:

- Precipitation of cardiac failure.
- Atrioventricular block.
- Constipation.

Other drugs not in this classification

These include:

- Digitalis (digoxin) – used for supraventricular arrhythmias, especially atrial fibrillation. It has a central effect, stimulating the vagus nerve resulting in partial atrioventricular block. This slows the ventricular beat and causes stronger contractions. It also inhibits Na^+/K^+ ATPase.

- Adenosine – used to terminate supraventricular tachycardias.
- Magnesium chloride – used for ventricular arrhythmias and to treat digoxin excess.
- Atropine – used to treat bradycardia. It acts by blocking parasympathetic effects on the heart.
- Adrenaline – used in cardiac arrest as a vasoconstrictor and to increase myocardial perfusion.
- Isoprenaline – used in the treatment of heart block while awaiting pacing.

Sicilian Gambit classification

In 1991, a group of basic and clinical investigators devised a new classification for anti-arrhythmic drugs. Anti-arrhythmic drugs fit awkwardly into the Vaughan-Williams classification because of their mixed actions. This new classification provides the best information available on the current anti-arrhythmic drugs based on their individual actions. This classification has taken over from the Vaughan-Williams classification. A spreadsheet of the actions of current medication has been published (Fig. 5.7).

Other treatments for arrhythmias

Non-medical management of arrhythmias should be considered for:

- New-onset arrhythmias.
- Failed medical therapy.
- Immediately life-threatening arrhythmias.

DC shock (cardioversion therapy)

Defibrillation is used to treat ventricular fibrillation, and cardioversion therapy is used to treat other serious arrhythmias. A defibrillator is used to give a shock to the heart through the skin. This should abolish the arrhythmia and allow the sinoatrial node to take back control of the heart's rhythm. Implantable cardiac defibrillators (ICDs) are available and can be implanted into the body. These ICD devices detect any arrhythmia that may occur, and act by either delivering a small shock to return the

heart to sinus rhythm, or by overdrive pacing, whereby the ventricle is paced rapidly out of the arrhythmia and then slowed back down to a normal rate. Triggered DC shock is the treatment of choice for broad QRS complex tachycardias. The shock must be synchronized and delivered on the S wave of the electrocardiogram.

Pacemaker

This is often used in sick sinus syndrome where there is disease of the sinus node (ischaemia, infarction or degeneration), leading to pauses in sinus node function or bradycardia. It is also used for complete heart block, Mobitz type 2 block (as this frequently progresses to complete heart block), suppression of atrial fibrillation and for malignant vasovagal syndrome. Pacemakers can be implanted into the body to control the heart rate. An electrode is placed in the right atrium and linked to a voltage generator. This artificial pacemaker is then set at a certain frequency such that it takes over the role of the sinoatrial node in generating cardiac depolarization.

If the atrium is fibrillating when there is heart block, a ventricular electrode is used. Heart block with intact atrial function requires a dual chamber pacemaker.

DISORDERS OF THE HEART VALVES

Heart valve disease produces two types of disorder: stenosis and regurgitation. Stenosis is an obstruction to the normal flow of blood, whereas regurgitation (incompetence or reflux) is a failure of preventing the backflow of blood. Both conditions can coexist in the same valve (e.g. mitral stenosis and regurgitation after rheumatic fever).

Valvular disease can be caused by direct leaflet damage or by valve ring damage, or it may be secondary to damage of the papillary muscles or chordae. Major causes of acquired valve disease are as follows:

- Mitral stenosis – can be caused by rheumatic fever.
- Mitral regurgitation – can be caused by rheumatic fever, mitral valve prolapse, papillary muscle dysfunction, or valve ring dilatation.

Fig. 5.7 Spreadsheet approach to the classification of drugs (A_1, adenosine receptor; I_f, inward background depolarizing current of pacemaker caused by Na^+ and Ca^{2+}, termed 'funny'; M_2, muscarinic receptor; Lidocaine, lignocaine). (Reproduced from Eur Heart J. Vol 17, March 1996. With permission of The European Society of Cardiology.)

Drug	Channels Na fast	med	slow	Ca	K	I_f	α	β	M_2	A_1	Pumps Na^+/K^+ ATPase	left ven-tricular function	sinus rate	extra-cardiac	PR interval	QRS width	JT interval
Lidocaine	□											→	→	▦			↓
Mexiletine	□											→	→				↓
Tocainide	□											→	→	■			↓
Moricizine	⊗											↓	→	□		↑	
Procainamide		✓			▦							↓	→	■	↑	↑	↑
Disopyramide		✓			▦				□			↓	→	▦	↑↓	↑	↑
Quinidine		✓			▦		□		□			→	↑	▦	↑↓	↑	↑
Propafenone		✓						▦				↓	↓	□	↑	↑	
Flecainide			✓		□							↓	→	□	↑	↑	
Encainide			✓									↓	→	□	↑	↑	
Bepridil	□			■	▦							↓		□			↑
Verapamil	□			■			▦					↓	↓	□	↑		
Diltiazem				▦								↓	↓	□	↑		
Bretylium				■			◐	◐				→	↓	□			↑
Sotalol				■				■				↓	↓	□	↑		↑
Amiodarone	□			■	□		▦	▦				→	↓	■		↑	↑
Alinidine				▦	■								↓	■			
Nadolol								■				↓	↓	□	↓		
Propranolol	□							■				↓	↓	□	↑		
Atropine									■			→	↑	▦	↓		
Adenosine										○			↓	□	↑		
Digoxin									○		■	↑	↓	■	↑		↓

relative potency of block: □ low ▦ moderate ■ high   ✓ = activated state blocker ○ = agonist ◐ = agonist/antagonist ⊗ = inactivated state blocker

- Aortic stenosis – can be caused by rheumatic fever or calcific degeneration of a normal or bicuspid valve.
- Aortic regurgitation – can be caused by rheumatic fever, aortic dilatation, or rheumatological disorders.

Degenerative valve disease
Calcific aortic stenosis

Calcific aortic stenosis accounts for 90% of acquired aortic stenosis. This is thought to be an age-related degeneration, more common in the very old (aged over 70 years). Congenital bicuspid aortic valves (usually the valves are tricuspid) occur in 1% of the population. These valves become calcified much earlier in life (from about 50 years of age).

Rigid calcified deposits occur on the sinuses of Valsalva, resulting in thick, immobile valve cusps with narrowing of the orifice. Left ventricular hypertrophy usually results. Intervention (usually in the form of valve replacement) is required if angina, syncope or heart failure result.

Mitral annular calcification

Mitral annular calcification produces mitral regurgitation because the valve ring does not contract properly during systole. The condition also causes mitral stenosis because the bulky deposits prevent opening of the valves. Mitral annular calcification occurs more commonly in the elderly. Mitral stenosis increases the risk of thrombosis within the left atrium with subsequent systemic thromboembolism.

Calcific deposits may interfere with the conduction pathway, leading to arrhythmias, and they may also be a focus for infective endocarditis.

Myxomatous degeneration of the mitral valve (mitral valve prolapse)

Myxomatous degeneration causes billowing or prolapse of the mitral valve during systole, leading to regurgitation. The condition occurs in 15% of patients aged over 70 years. Cusps are thickened because of myxomatous (mucoid) deposition and fibrosis. Usually, this condition is asymptomatic except for a midsystolic click; an audible late systolic murmur indicates regurgitation. In severe disease, the chordae tendineae can rupture causing sudden, severe regurgitation.

Rheumatic heart disease

Rheumatic heart disease is a consequence of rheumatic fever that may have occurred many years previously. The acute process can leave the valves scarred and deformed, causing chronic rheumatic heart disease. This occurs if the onset of acute rheumatic fever is in early childhood and severe, or in chronic rheumatic fever.

Acute rheumatic fever

Acute rheumatic fever is an inflammatory disease caused by an autoimmune reaction initiated by infection with group A streptococci, usually in the throat. It mostly affects children aged 5–15 years. Now rare in the UK (occurring in 0.01% of children), it is common in the Middle East, Eastern Europe, Far East, and South America.

It affects the heart, skin, joints, and central nervous system. The Duckett Jones criteria for diagnosis include:

- Carditis involving all three layers (pancarditis).
- Sydenham's chorea (St Vitus dance; rapid, involuntary purposeless movements).
- Polyarthritis affecting the large joints.
- Erythema marginatum (macular rash with erythematous edge).
- Subcutaneous nodules.

Fever, arthralgia, and leucocytosis also commonly occur.

Carditis consists of granulomatous lesions with a central necrotic area (Aschoff nodule). Initially, there are macrophages, lymphocytes, and plasma cells, but these are replaced by fibrous scar tissue. On the valve, Aschoff nodules give rise to small vegetations (verrucae) of platelets and fibrin, which look like beads. Commonly, this affects the mitral valve (65%) or the mitral and aortic valves (25%). Recurrence is common if persistent carditis is present.

Chronic rheumatic fever

Chronic rheumatic fever is repeated attacks of rheumatic fever leading to chronic rheumatic heart disease, occurring in over half the patients with rheumatic carditis. This leads to commissural fusion, shortening/thickening of the chordae, and cusp fibrosis – the so-called fish-mouth or button-hole mitral valve deformity. Secondary changes in the heart occur as a result of:

- Mitral stenosis and regurgitation – leads to left atrial hypertrophy, pulmonary hypertension, atrial fibrillation, and thrombosis.
- Aortic stenosis – leads to left ventricular hypertrophy and arrhythmia.
- Aortic regurgitation – leads to left ventricular hypertrophy and dilatation.

Infective endocarditis

Infective endocarditis is an infection of the endocardium or vascular endothelium, usually involving the heart valves. Previously, endocarditis was classified as acute or subacute (Fig. 5.8); now it is classified according to the causative organism. The incidence is 6–7 per 100,000 in the UK, but it is more common in developing countries.

Infective endocarditis occurs more commonly on valves that have been previously damaged or are congenitally abnormal. Inflammation of the valve causes destruction and scarring.

Vegetations (consisting of fibrin, platelets, and the infecting organism) usually arise on the valves.

Causative agents include:

- *Streptococcus viridans* – subacute; common after dental procedures, tonsillectomy, or bronchoscopy.
- *Staphylococcus aureus* – acute; common in patients with indwelling catheters and intravenous drug users.
- *Enterococcus faecalis* – common in patients with pelvic infections or after having pelvic surgery.
- *Coxiella burnetti* (Q fever) – subacute.
- *Staphylococcus epidermidis, Aspergillus, Candida, Brucella, Histoplasma* – common in drug addicts and patients with prosthetic heart valves.

Sequelae of infective endocarditis include:

- Acute valve incompetence.
- Emboli to spleen, kidneys, and brain.
- Glomerulonephritis and renal failure.

Non-infective endocarditis

There are two main causes of non-infective endocarditis, both of which are very rare:

- Marantic endocarditis.
- Libman–Sacks disease (endocarditis of systemic lupus erythematosus).

Carcinoid heart disease

Argentaffinomas (tumours of the argentaffin cells of the intestine) produce physiologically active substances [e.g. 5-hydroxytryptamine (serotonin), bradykinin, prostaglandins], which cause thickening of the tricuspid and pulmonary valve and parts of the right ventricle. The left side is usually unaffected.

DISEASES OF THE MYOCARDIUM

Myocardial disease can be categorized as either a cardiomyopathy or a specific disease of heart muscle:

- A cardiomyopathy is any chronic disease affecting the muscle of the heart for which the cause is unknown (i.e. idiopathic, primary).
- Specific heart muscle disease is a heart muscle disease for which the cause is known or associated with other disorders.

Myocardial dysfunction may also be a result of:

- Congenital heart disease.
- Hypertension.
- Ischaemia.

Acute compared with subacute manifestations of infective endocarditis		
Features	Acute	Subacute
Virulence of organism	High	Moderate or low
State of valve before infection	Normal	Injured or abnormal
Type of infection	Necrotizing and invasive	Less destructive
Macroscopic vegetations	Larger and may cause emboli	Small to large
Presentation	Fever, rigors, malaise, splenomegaly, heart murmur	Low-grade fever, weight loss, flu-like syndrome, heart murmur
Course	Death occurs in 50% within days	Protracted course; often less fatal

Fig. 5.8 Acute compared with subacute manifestations of infective endocarditis.

- Valve disease.
- Pericardial disease.

Myocarditis is inflammation of the myocardium, and it is one of the main functional classes of specific heart muscle disease.

Cardiomyopathy and neoplastic heart disease are, in comparison to ischaemic heart disease, very rare. It is important to bear this in mind when learning about conditions which affect the cardiovascular system.

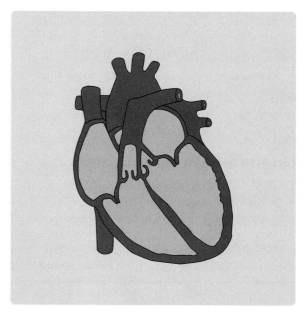

Fig. 5.9 A normal heart for comparison with the cardiomyopathic hearts shown in Figs 5.10–5.12.

Cardiomyopathy

Cardiomyopathy is often functionally classified according to presentation into the following diseases:

- Dilated (congestive) cardiomyopathy (85%) – with dilated left ventricle and impaired systolic function.
- Hypertrophic (obstructive) cardiomyopathy (10%) – hypertrophy of ventricles, especially the interventricular septum; reduced diastolic filling.
- Restrictive cardiomyopathy (5%) – decreased ventricular compliance restricts ventricular filling.

Dilated cardiomyopathy

In contrast to the normal heart (Fig. 5.9), dilated cardiomyopathy causes dilated ventricles and poor contraction (Fig. 5.10). Its prevalence is 0.2%.
Pathogenic factors include:

- Genetic defect.
- Alcohol toxicity.
- Postviral myocarditis – some myocarditis progresses to ventricular dilatation.
- Peripartum – may be caused by physiological, pathological or metabolic changes in pregnancy.

Other associations include:

- Cardiovascular disease (e.g. ischaemia, hypertension).
- Systemic disease (e.g. sarcoidosis, systemic lupus erythematosus, haemochromatosis).

Fig. 5.10 Dilated cardiomyopathy. The ventricles are thin and dilated. Compare with Fig. 5.9.

- Neuromuscular disease (e.g. muscular dystrophy, Friedreich's ataxia).
- Haemochromatosis.
- Glycogen storage disorder.
- Primary heart muscle disease (e.g. amyloidosis).
- Drug therapy: cytotoxic drugs (e.g. cyclophosphamide).

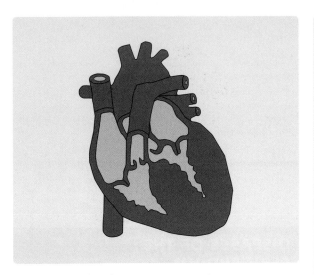

Fig. 5.11 Hypertrophic cardiomyopathy. There is an increase in ventricular mass. Compare with Fig. 5.9.

The morphology of dilated cardiomyopathy is as follows:

- Cardiomegaly with dilated thin walls in all chambers.
- Irregular myocyte hypertrophy and fibrosis.

Dilated cardiomyopathy can cause heart failure, arrhythmia, and emboli. Mortality is 40% within 2 years.

Hypertrophic (obstructive) cardiomyopathy

Hypertrophic cardiomyopathy (HOCM) (Fig. 5.11) is characterized by hypertrophy of the ventricles and septum; often it is asymmetrical. The disease causes distorted contraction and abnormal mitral valve movement. It is more common in young adults, and 50% of cases are inherited (autosomal dominant). The morphology of the hypertrophic cardiomyopathy is as follows:

- Asymmetrical septal hypertrophy.
- Left ventricular cavity is banana-like.
- Myofibre hypertrophy and disarray.
- Patchy fibrosis.

Hypertrophic cardiomyopathy can also cause dyspnoea, angina, syncope, and sudden death. Characteristic findings include a fourth heart sound, jerky pulse, and systolic murmur. The course of the disease is very variable; most patients remain unaffected for years.

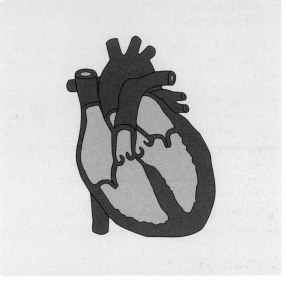

Fig. 5.12 Restrictive cardiomyopathy. The heart is of normal size, but the ventricles are stiff. Compare with Fig. 5.9.

Restrictive cardiomyopathy

Restrictive cardiomyopathy (Fig. 5.12) is a stiffening of the myocardium with restricted ventricular filling. It is often associated with:

- Amyloidosis – most common form in the Western world.
- Endomyocardial fibrosis – children and young adults in Africa.
- Loeffler's endocarditis – found in temperate climates.

There is interstitial myocardial fibrosis (associated with eosinophilia in the latter two conditions). Dyspnoea, fatigue, and emboli may be the presenting features. Symptoms are often similar to those seen in constrictive pericarditis.

Specific disease of the myocardium

Myocarditis

Myocarditis is inflammation of the myocardium. Causes include:

- Infection – viruses (coxsackie, influenza, rubella, echovirus, polio); bacteria (*Corynebacterium* – diphtheria, *Rickettsia*, *Chlamydia*); protozoa (*Trypanosoma cruzi* –

Chagas' disease, *Toxoplasma gondii*); fungi (*Candida*).

- Immune-mediated reactions – after infections (viral or rheumatic fever); systemic lupus erythematosus; transplant rejection; chemicals, radiation and drugs (chloroquine, methyldopa, lead poisoning).
- Idiopathic causes – sarcoidosis, giant cell myocarditis.

The morphology of myocarditis is as follows:

- Loose myocardial tissue with dilatation in all four chambers.
- Haemorrhagic mottling.
- Mural thrombi.
- Inflammatory infiltrate with focal myocyte necrosis and fibrosis.

Patients present with fever, dyspnoea, angina, arrhythmia, and heart failure; the presentation is similar to myocardial infarction but often less acute.

Other diseases

Other specific heart muscle diseases are generally associated with cardiotoxic agents, which cause myocyte swelling, fatty change, and cell lysis. Fibrosis and scarring usually replace the focal lesions.

The various causes are explained below.

Alcohol
Alcohol causes a similar morphology to dilated cardiomyopathy. It may be associated with thiamine deficiency.

Adriamycin (doxorubicin) and other drugs
These cytotoxic drugs in toxic levels cause oxidation of the myocyte membranes, causing a similar morphology to dilated cardiomyopathy.

Catecholamines
Either exogenous (e.g. administered adrenaline) or endogenous (e.g. in phaeochromocytoma) catecholamines can cause tachycardia and vasoconstriction, leading to patchy ischaemic necrosis. This leads to a dilated cardiomyopathy. Cocaine may have a similar effect as it stops noradrenaline uptake.

Peripartum state
A dilated heart is found several months before and after delivery. The mechanism for this is uncertain, but it may include hypertension, volume overload, nutritional deficiency, immune reaction, or metabolic dysfunction. In 50% of these patients, function is restored several months later.

Amyloidosis
Amyloidosis may be systemic or isolated. It may induce arrhythmia or restrictive cardiomyopathy.

Iron overload
Patients with iron overload present with a dilated cardiomyopathy. This is often found in hereditary haemochromatosis and haemosiderosis (excess blood transfusion).

DISEASES OF THE PERICARDIUM

Fluid accumulation in the pericardial sac

Normally, the pericardial sac contains 50 mL of serous fluid. Its functions include:

- Lubrication.
- Prevention of sudden deformation or dislocation.
- A barrier to the spread of infection.

Slow effusions allow greater volumes to accumulate before reaching the clinical threshold.

Pericardial effusion

A pericardial effusion:

- Is an accumulation of fluid in the pericardial cavity.
- Can be caused by any condition causing pericarditis.
- Can usually be morphologically classified as serous, serosanguinous, or chylous.

The effusion collects in the closed cavity and causes distension. When the pericardium cannot distend any more, abnormally high pressures build up and cardiac tamponade results (impaired ventricular filling leading to loss of cardiac output).

Serous
In a serous effusion, there is a smooth glistening serosa. Fluid accumulates slowly. The effusion is caused by heart failure and hypoproteinaemia.

Serosanguinous

These effusions are usually caused by blunt chest trauma, infections such as tuberculosis or pneumonia, and malignant infiltration of the pericardium.

Chylous

Chylous effusions are caused by lymphatic obstruction.

Haemopericardium

Haemopericardium is the accumulation of blood in the pericardial sac. It is caused by:

- Myocardial rupture after a myocardial infarction.
- Rupture of the intrapericardial aorta.
- Dissecting aortic aneurysm.
- Haemorrhage from an abscess or tumour.
- Trauma.

If the accumulation of blood is greater than 200–300 mL, cardiac tamponade can result.

Clinical features of cardiac tamponade are those of heart failure, including a raised jugular venous pressure, Kussmaul's sign, exaggerated pulsus paradoxus, soft heart sounds, and a non-palpable apex beat. If a frictional rub was present, it may be quieter than before as the fluid separates the parietal and visceral pericardium.

Investigation and treatment

An echocardiogram is the best method for diagnosing a pericardial effusion. The effusion must be tapped (pericardiocentesis) if it severely compromises the circulation (i.e. when the effusion develops rapidly). Reaccumulation occurs with purulent, tuberculous, and malignant effusions.

Pericarditis

Pericarditis is an inflammation of the pericardium leading to sharp substernal chest pain that radiates to the back, and that is aggravated by movement and respiration. Common causes are listed in Fig. 5.13.

Acute pericarditis

Commonly, acute pericarditis is caused by an acute viral (coxsackie) infection or a myocardial infarction. Morphologically acute pericarditis can be separated into:

Common causes of pericarditis	
Cause	Pathology
Viral (coxsackievirus)	Fibrinous
Myocardial infarction	Fibrinous and may lead to fibrous adhesions
Uraemia	Fibrinous
Carcinoma (metastatic spread, often from the lung)	Serous or haemorrhagic
Connective tissue disease (rheumatic fever)	Fibrinous
Bacterial	Purulent
Tuberculosis	Caseous
After cardiac surgery	Fibrinous
Dressler's syndrome (after a myocardial infarction)	Autoimmune

Fig. 5.13 Common causes of pericarditis.

- Serous – slowly accumulating serous exudate with inflammatory cells.
- Fibrinous/serofibrinous – most common, may resolve completely or leave adhesions.
- Suppurative (purulent) – bacterial/fungal infection with pus; may produce constrictive pericarditis.
- Haemorrhagic – blood exudate with fibrin or pus; may calcify.
- Caseous – leads to constrictive pericarditis; caused by tuberculosis.

Chronic pericarditis

Healing of pericarditis can result in complete resolution, thick plaques, or adhesions.

Adhesive pericarditis

In adhesive pericarditis, the parietal pericardium becomes attached to the mediastinum and the pericardial sac no longer exists. The heart dilates and hypertrophies.

Constrictive pericarditis

In constrictive pericarditis, there is a thick, fibrous, often calcified pericardial sac that encases the heart, limiting cardiac filling and reducing cardiac output. Symptoms of heart failure result.

Rheumatic disease of the pericardium

Pericarditis occurs in 30% of people with severe chronic rheumatoid arthritis. Granulomas may lead to fibrous adhesions, causing constrictive pericarditis.

CONGENITAL ABNORMALITIES OF THE HEART

Congenital heart defects have an incidence of 6–8 per 1000 live-born infants. They may present in the first year of life or remain asymptomatic for life.

Left-to-right shunts

Left-to-right shunts very rarely cause cyanosis.

Atrial septal defect

An atrial septal defect (ASD) is caused by a failure of proper closure of the foramen ovale or by a defect in the septum secundum (see p. 15). Blood moves from the left atrium into the right atrium because of the pressure difference (Fig. 5.14). Atrial septal defects make up 10% of all congenital heart defects. Frequently, the child is asymptomatic, but clinical features can include:

- Recurrent chest infections, heart failure, and arrhythmias.
- Fixed, widely split second heart sound.
- Ejection systolic murmur, best heard in the third intercostal space, produced by increased flow across the pulmonary valve (left-to-right shunt).

Electrocardiography, chest radiography, and echocardiography will confirm the diagnosis. In children with symptoms, treatment is by a catheter-delivered device or surgery.

Ventricular septal defect

A ventricular septal defect (VSD) is a failure of fusion of the interventricular septum or endocardial cushions (Fig. 5.15). Blood shunts through a hole in the interventricular septum.

Ventricular septal defects make up 30% of all congenital heart lesions. The patient may be asymptomatic, but clinical features can include:

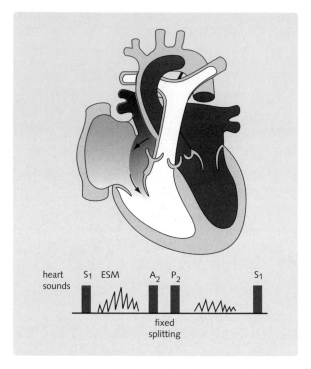

Fig. 5.14 Atrial septal defect (S_1, first heart sound from closure of mitral and tricuspid valves; A_2, heart sound from closure of aortic valve; ESM, ejection systolic murmur; P_2, heart sound from closure of pulmonary valve). (Courtesy of Lissauer T, Clayden G. Illustrated textbook of paediatrics, 2nd edn. London: Mosby, 2001.)

- Heart failure, failure to thrive, recurrent chest infections.
- Palpable parasternal thrill.
- Loud pansystolic murmur at lower left sternal edge.

Electrocardiography, echocardiography, and chest radiography will confirm the diagnosis.

Most ventricular septal defects will close spontaneously within the first 2 years of life. However, 10% will require drug therapy (for heart failure) or surgery.

If there is a large left-to-right shunt, there will be a great deal of blood entering the right ventricle and pulmonary circulation, causing pulmonary hypertension. Eventually, the pulmonary hypertension will cause irreversible damage to the pulmonary vasculature. This will cause right ventricular hypertrophy, which may eventually lead to reversal of the shunt from right to left. This phenomenon is irreversible and is known as Eisenmenger's syndrome. It frequently leads to cyanosis (Fig. 5.16).

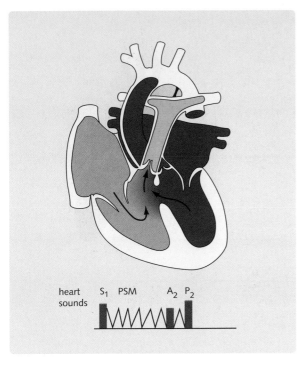

Fig. 5.15 Ventricular septal defect (S_1, first heart sound from closure of mitral and tricuspid valves; A_2, heart sound from closure of aortic valve; PSM, pansystolic murmur; P_2, heart sound from closure of pulmonary valve). (Courtesy of Lissauer T, Clayden G. Illustrated textbook of paediatrics, 2nd edn. London: Mosby, 2001.)

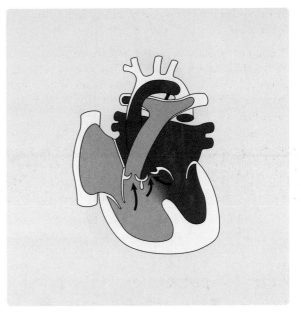

Fig. 5.16 Eisenmenger's syndrome. The shunt has reversed (and now goes from right to left). Less blood now goes into the pulmonary trunk and the patient becomes cyanosed. (Courtesy of Lissauer T, Clayden G. Illustrated textbook of paediatrics, 2nd edn. London: Mosby, 2001.)

Other large left-to-right shunts (e.g. atrial septal defects or patent ductus arteriosus) can also lead to Eisenmenger's syndrome.

Patent ductus arteriosus

Patent ductus arteriosus is caused by an open ductus arteriosus, which allows the communication of blood between the systemic and pulmonary circulations (Fig. 5.17). It accounts for 10% of all congenital heart defects.

There is a continuous murmur beneath the left clavicle and a collapsing pulse.

Echocardiography is the most useful investigation.

In preterm infants, the duct will ultimately close, but it can be closed with indomethacin (inhibits prostaglandin production), or it may require closure with a catheter-delivered device.

Infective endocarditis may result if the duct never closes.

When considering congenital disorders of the heart, it is important to visualize the pressure changes that occur in the cardiac cycle in order to work out which shunting mechanism and murmur occurs with each defect. For example, in a ventricular septal defect the left ventricular pressure is greater than the right because of its larger muscle mass, so, therefore, blood is going to flow from left to right. As this shunt occurs throughout systole a pansystolic murmur occurs. Cyanosis does not occur unless deoxygenated blood 'dilutes' oxygenated blood before entering the systemic circulation.

Atrioventricular septal defect

An atrioventricular septal defect (AVSD) results from failure of the superior and inferior endocardial cushions to fuse (Fig. 5.18). This is pathognomonic of Down syndrome. Surgical repair is complex and hazardous.

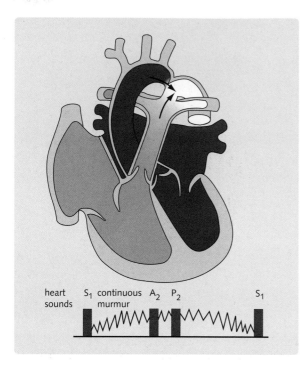

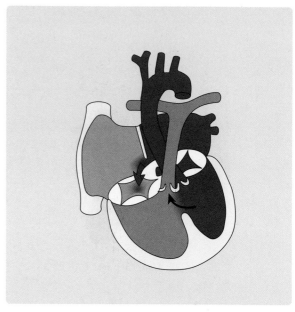

Fig. 5.17 Patent ductus arteriosus. This is often found with coarctation of the aorta (shown). It allows mixing of systemic and pulmonary blood. Movement of blood within the ductus can occur in both directions depending upon the relative pressures in the aorta and the pulmonary trunk (S_1, first heart sound from closure of mitral and tricuspid valves; A_2, heart sound from closure of aortic valve; P_2, heart sound from closure of pulmonary valve). (Courtesy of Lissauer T, Clayden G. Illustrated textbook of paediatrics, 2nd edn. London: Mosby, 2001.)

Fig. 5.18 Atrioventricular septal defect (AVSD). There is very little separation between the atria and ventricles. (Courtesy of Lissauer T, Clayden G. Illustrated textbook of paediatrics, 2nd edn. London: Mosby, 2001.)

Right-to-left shunts

Right-to-left shunts commonly cause cyanosis.

Tetralogy of Fallot

Tetralogy of Fallot (Fig. 5.19) is a combination of:

- Large ventricular septal defect.
- Infundibular pulmonary stenosis (responsible for the audible murmur).
- Right ventricular hypertrophy.
- Aorta overriding the interventricular septum.

The tetralogy occurs in 6% of children with heart defects. Severe cyanosis with hypercyanotic episodes may result. A loud ejection systolic murmur is heard in the third left intercostal space, and finger clubbing may develop. Corrective

surgery is required, which can be started at 4–6 months of age.

Transposition of the great arteries

Transposition of the great arteries occurs when the truncoconal septum develops, but it does not spiral (Fig. 5.20). The left ventricle pumps blood into the pulmonary trunk and the right ventricle pumps blood into the aorta. There is usually also an atrial septal defect, ventricular septal defect, or patent ductus arteriosus to allow blood to mix, otherwise this would be incompatible with life.

Transposition of the great arteries occurs in 4% of cardiac defects. Severe cyanosis may result. There may be finger clubbing and numerous murmurs. The definitive treatment is an arterial switch procedure.

Persistent truncus arteriosus

The truncoconal septum fails to form, leading to a common outflow tract for both ventricles. There is also a ventricular septal defect in this very rare condition.

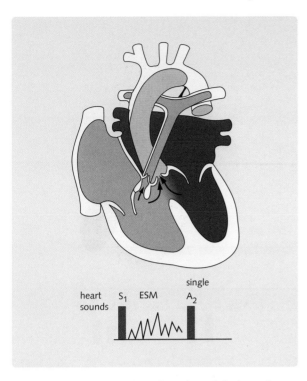

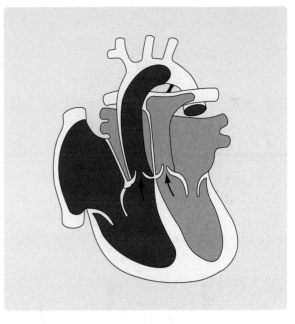

Fig. 5.19 Tetralogy of Fallot. The right-to-left shunt that results causes cyanosis (S_1, first heart sound from closure of mitral and tricuspid valves; A_2, heart sound from closure of aortic valve; ESM, ejection systolic murmur). (Courtesy of Lissauer T, Clayden G. Illustrated textbook of paediatrics, 2nd edn. London: Mosby, 2001.)

Fig. 5.20 Transposition of the great arteries. This is incompatible with life without a ventricular (VSD) or atrial septal defect (ASD) or a patent ductus arteriosus. (Courtesy of Lissauer T, Clayden G. Illustrated textbook of paediatrics, 2nd edn. London: Mosby, 2001.)

Tricuspid atresia

In tricuspid atresia, there is an absence of the tricuspid valve, causing poor pulmonary circulation. The neonate has a duct-dependent circulation (i.e. other communications are needed between the arterial and venous systems to prevent serious cyanosis). Surgery is required to place a tricuspid valve.

Obstructive congenital defects

Coarctation of the aorta

Coarctation of the aorta is a narrowing of the aorta around the area of the ductus arteriosus (Fig. 5.21). It is frequently associated with a ventricular septal defect and a bicuspid aortic valve. Coarctation occurs in 7% of children with congenital heart defects. The diagnosis can be made from weak or absent femoral pulses. There is also an ejection sys-

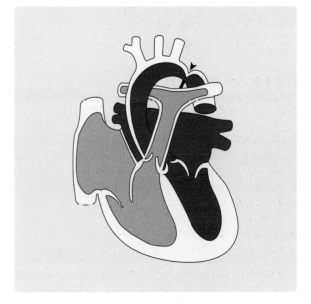

Fig. 5.21 Coarctation of the aorta, causing stenosis. (Courtesy of Lissauer T, Clayden G. Illustrated textbook of paediatrics, 2nd edn. London: Mosby, 2001.)

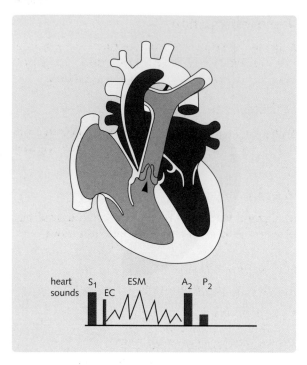

Fig. 5.22 Pulmonary stenosis (S$_1$, first heart sound from closure of mitral and tricuspid valves; A$_2$, heart sound from closure of aortic valve; EC, ejection click; ESM, ejection systolic murmur; P$_2$, heart sound from closure of pulmonary valve). (Courtesy of Lissauer T, Clayden G. Illustrated textbook of paediatrics, 2nd edn. London: Mosby, 2001.)

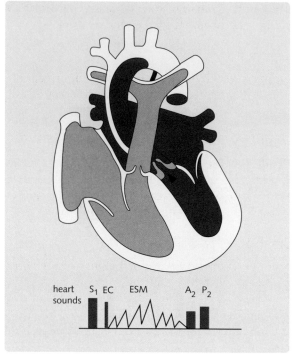

Fig. 5.23 Aortic stenosis (S$_1$, first heart sound from closure of mitral and tricuspid valves; A$_2$, heart sound from closure of aortic valve; EC, ejection click; ESM, ejection systolic murmur; P$_2$, heart sound from closure of pulmonary valve). (Courtesy of Lissauer T, Clayden G. Illustrated textbook of paediatrics, 2nd edn. London: Mosby, 2001.)

tolic murmur heard at the back. Surgery is required to correct the defect.

Pulmonary stenosis with intact interventricular septum

Of those children with heart defects, 7% present with a stenosis of the pulmonary valve (Fig. 5.22); most are asymptomatic. An ejection systolic murmur and ejection click may be heard. Treatment is indicated when right ventricular hypertrophy occurs or the stenosis worsens.

Aortic stenosis

Stenosis of the aortic valve occurs in 6% of neonates with heart defects (Fig. 5.23). Usually there is associated mitral stenosis and coarctation of the aorta. There may be heart failure, syncope, and chest pain. Clinical features also include slow-rising pulses, an ejection click, and ejection systolic murmur. Eventually valve replacement is necessary.

NEOPLASTIC HEART DISEASE

Primary cardiac tumours

Primary cardiac tumours include myxoma, lipoma, papillary fibroelastoma, rhabdomyoma and sarcoma. They are extremely rare.

Myxoma

Myxomas account for 25% of primary cardiac tumours. Presentation can be at any age, but mostly it occurs in adults; 75% of myxomas occur in the left atrium. They can be polyploid or pedunculated masses, arising from undifferentiated connective tissue in the subendocardial layer. If pedunculated, the tumour mass may have limited movement within the heart chamber, sufficient to periodically occlude cardiac outflow (ball-valve obstruction). Of patients with myxoma, 50% show signs and symptoms of mitral valve disease. Myxomatous masses can fragment and produce emboli.

Lipoma

Lipomas usually occur in the interatrial septum. They are well circumscribed, poorly encapsulated adipose tissue.

Papillary fibroelastoma

Papillary fibroelastomas are filamentous projections found in right-sided valves in children and left-sided valves in adults. They are composed of connective tissue with smooth muscle and fibroblasts.

Rhabdomyoma

Many rhabdomyomas occur in neonates, causing stillbirth or death in the first few days of life. They are often multiple, and they arise from cardiac muscle. They have strands in the cytoplasm radiating out of the nucleus, and so they are called spider cells.

Sarcoma

Malignant tumours include rhabdomyosarcomas and angiosarcomas.

Cardiovascular effects of neoplastic disease

Metastases

Metastases that develop in the myocardium are usually from bronchial carcinomas or malignant melanomas. They are much more common than primary tumours of cardiac tissue.

Vessel obstruction

A tumour can obstruct neighbouring vessels by local invasion into vessel walls, compression by growth outside the vessel, and by producing emboli.

Emboli

Tumours can fragment and send off emboli that will impact in a vessel (e.g. a tumour in the leg may cause a pulmonary embolus).

Haemorrhage

Malignant tumours on mucosa can ulcerate and bleed. Bleeding can also occur into a tumour.

Circulating factors

Circulating factors can lead to:

- Non-bacterial thrombotic endocarditis.
- Carcinoid heart disease.
- Myeloma-associated amyloidosis.
- Phaeochromocytoma-associated heart disease.

Iatrogenic effects of therapy

There are many unwanted effects of therapy of neoplastic disease. Radiotherapy causes lethargy, appetite loss, and rashes, for example. Chemotherapy causes nausea, vomiting, alopecia, and marrow suppression. Each modality and substance has its own specific side effects. Surgical therapy can be risky and complicated, especially as some tissues are highly vascularized. However, there are few general iatrogenic effects that affect the cardiovascular system.

The cardiovascular system in disease – diseases of the vessels

Objectives

You should be able to:

- Understand the pathological basis of arteriosclerosis and atherosclerosis.
- Define shock and list the main causes.
- Outline the risk factors for and complications of hypertension.
- Describe how lipids are transported and metabolized, and how this may be modified with drugs.
- Describe the main causes and types of aneurysms.
- Describe the various classifications of the vasculitides.
- Describe the common congenital abnormalities of the vessels.
- Outline the various benign and malignant lesions which affect the vessels.
- Recall the risk factors for varicose veins and deep venous thrombosis.
- Understand the causes of lymphoedema and lymphangitis and how they arise.

ARTERIOSCLEROSIS AND ATHEROSCLEROSIS

Definitions and concepts

Arteriosclerosis is a term used to describe hardening and thickening of arteries. This reduces their elastic properties.

Atherosclerosis is one of the processes that leads to arteriosclerosis, and is the main cause of both ischaemic heart disease (see p. 77) and peripheral vascular disease (see p. 108). It involves the formation of atheroma, an accumulation of lipid plaques, within the walls of a vessel.

Arteriosclerosis of small arteries and arterioles is termed arteriolosclerosis, and is predominantly caused by hypertension.

There are three main types of arteriosclerosis:

- Atherosclerosis.
- Arteriolosclerosis.
- Monckeberg's calcific medial sclerosis.

Consequences of arteriosclerosis

Arteriosclerosis results in a reduced arterial lumen with a consequent reduction in end-organ perfusion. Furthermore, due to the loss of elasticity, rupture is more likely. There is also a predisposition to thrombus formation.

Atherosclerosis

It has been said that every adult in the Western world has some degree of atheroma in their arteries. Atherosclerosis and its complications are the main cause of mortality (over 50%) in the Western world.

Risk factors

Risk factors for atherosclerosis include constitutional factors such as:

- Age. Increased age increases the number and severity of lesions.
- Male sex. Men are affected to a much greater extent than women, until the menopause when the incidence in women increases, but men continue to be predominantly affected.
- Genetic predisposition.

Strong risk factors for atherosclerosis are:

- Smoking.
- Hypertension.
- Diabetes mellitus (see below).
- Hyperlipidaemia. It is directly related to levels of cholesterol and LDL. HDL levels are protective.

Other factors involved in the development of atherosclerosis are:

Fig. 6.1 Stages in the formation of an atheromatous plaque. (A) Damage to the endothelium. Chronic or repeated endothelial cell (EC) injury occurs, leading to metabolic dysfunction and structural changes. EC have a major role in actively preventing thrombus formation. Damage activates EC, upregulating inflammatory adhesion molecules (e.g. ICAM-1) and promoting monocyte and platelet adhesion. Injury also increases permeability to lipids and low-density lipoprotein (LDL), allowing movement into the intima. (B) Formation of a fatty streak. Monocytes adhere to the endothelium, migrate into the intima and become macrophages. There, they take up the LDL and become foam cells as they cannot degrade lipids. Local oxidation of LDL aids uptake by, and is chemotactic for, macrophages. Platelets adhere to activated endothelial cells or areas of denuded matrix. Activated platelets, activated EC and macrophages release platelet-derived growth factor (PDGF) and induce smooth muscle migration into the intima. (C) Development of lipid plaque. Smooth muscle proliferation and an increase in extracellular matrix occur in the intima. Smooth muscle cells also take up LDL and form foam cells. Greater macrophage infiltration takes place. Lipid may also be released free into the intima. Macrophages contribute many other factors (e.g. superoxide, proteases) that increase the damage. (D) Complicated plaques. As the lesion develops, pressure causes the media to atrophy and the muscle to be replaced by collagen. A fibrous cap of collagen forms on top. There is increased free lipid in the intima. The endothelium becomes fragile and ulcerates, leading to further platelet aggregation and thrombus formation.

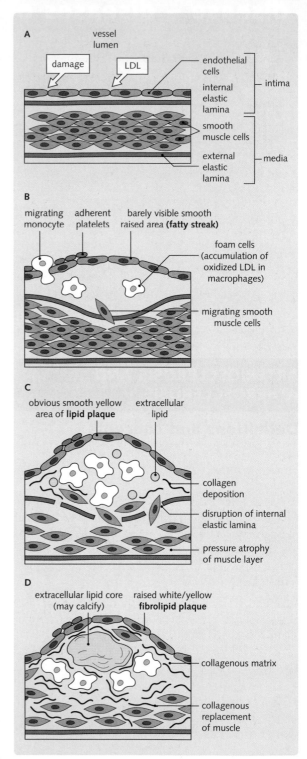

- Exercise – decreases the incidence of coronary heart disease; however, whether it prevents atheroma formation is unclear.
- Obesity – increases mortality, but this may only be a reflection of diet and lipid profile.
- Diet – decreased saturated fat intake has a beneficial effect, as may antioxidants (e.g. vitamin E in red wine).
- Stress and personality – certain highly stressed and type A personalities (anxious, moody and prone to worry) may have an increased tendency to atherosclerosis and coronary heart disease.

Pathogenesis

Atherosclerosis generally affects medium to large arteries. It is characterized by lipid deposition in the intima, with smooth muscle and matrix proliferation combining to produce a fibrous plaque that protrudes into the lumen (Fig. 6.1). The lesions tend to be focal, patchy, and not involve the whole circumference of the vessel.

Other theories of pathogenesis include:

- Prostaglandins. The balance between prostacyclin and thromboxane has an influence on thrombus formation and, because fibrin and platelets are important components of atheromatous lesions, this must have a strong influence on pathogenesis.
- Thrombosis is the primary event that builds up in layers and organizes to form atheromatous plaques.
- Neoplasia. An abnormal proliferation of smooth muscle occurs, caused by some as yet unidentified factor that produces uncontrolled growth.

Atherosclerosis is primarily an inflammatory process, and it is asymptomatic until it produces:

- Narrowing of the lumen – sufficient narrowing of the vessel produces symptoms of ischaemia (e.g. intermittent claudication, angina or gangrene).
- Sudden occlusion – caused by plaque rupture followed by thrombosis (e.g. in myocardial infarction).
- Emboli – these may impact in other vessels (e.g. stroke).
- Aneurysms – resulting from wall weakening.

Atheroma is a disease of the intima.

Treatment

The majority of research has looked at ways of reducing ischaemic heart disease by treating risk factors; it is not known what effect this has on the progress of atherosclerosis, but indirectly the following treatments have been used:

- Dietary control (reduced fat and sugar intake; increased amounts of fresh fruit and vegetables).
- Regular exercise and change in life-style (decrease stress).
- Stopping smoking.
- Cholesterol-lowering drugs (e.g. statins).
- Adequate blood pressure control.
- Optimal control of diabetes.

- Anti-platelet agents (e.g. aspirin and clopidogrel).

Monckeberg's medial calcific sclerosis

This is an idiopathic, degenerative disease of the elderly (aged over 50 years) characterized by focal calcifications in the media of small- and medium-sized arteries.

The femoral, tibial, radial and ulnar arteries are predominantly involved. There is little or no inflammation, and usually the calcifications do not cause either obstructions or symptoms. There is an increase in pulse pressure (isolated systolic hypertension) caused by loss of elasticity in the arteries.

Effects of diabetes mellitus on vessels

Diabetes mellitus causes a range of serious vascular complications, the severity of which is directly related to blood glucose levels. Intensive control of blood glucose (monitored long term by levels of glycosylated haemoglobin, HbA_{1C}), and treatment with ACE inhibitors can minimize these risks. Complications include:

- Microangiopathy.
- Hyaline arteriosclerosis.
- Atherosclerosis.

Type I diabetes is predominantly associated with small vessel disease (e.g. retinopathy, nephropathy, neuropathy), while type II predominantly causes large vessel disease (e.g. ischaemic heart disease and peripheral vascular disease).

Microangiopathy

Microangiopathy is diffuse thickening of the basement membranes of capillaries; paradoxically, however, they become more permeable, especially to plasma proteins. This results in specific organ damage:

- Nephropathy – glomerular involvement leads to microalbuminuria and can progress to renal failure.
- Retinopathy – degenerative changes include maculopathy and cataracts.
- Neuropathy – peripheral nerves, especially those in the lower leg, are most susceptible.

These phenomena are related to hyperglycaemia and the formation of advanced glycosylation end products.

Hyaline arteriosclerosis

Hyaline arteriosclerosis is more prevalent and more severe in patients with diabetes mellitus.

Atherosclerosis

Atherosclerosis begins early during the onset of diabetes mellitus. Complicated plaques become more numerous and severe. Contributing factors include:

- Associated hyperlipidaemia and decreased HDL.
- Glycosylation of LDL and its cross-linking with collagen.
- Increased platelet adhesion caused by obesity and hypertension.

Peripheral vascular disease

Atherosclerosis and diabetes related vessel damage may commonly occur in the lower limbs. The superficial femoral artery is most commonly targeted, although the aorta, iliac and common femoral arteries may also be involved.

The most common presentation is with intermittent claudication, i.e. pain brought on by walking as the muscles become ischaemic which is relieved by rest. Treatment at this stage involves modification of cardiovascular risk factors, smoking cessation being paramount. Continuing to exercise through the pain will help to develop a collateral circulation, improving blood supply to the lower limb, and should be encouraged.

Should the ischaemia worsen, ulceration and gangrene may occur (see p. 161). Critical ischaemia, i.e. pain at rest, should be treated either with a surgical bypass procedure (Fig. 6.2), or angioplasty. If the ischaemia is so severe that the limb becomes

Fig. 6.2 Bypass procedures in peripheral vascular disease.

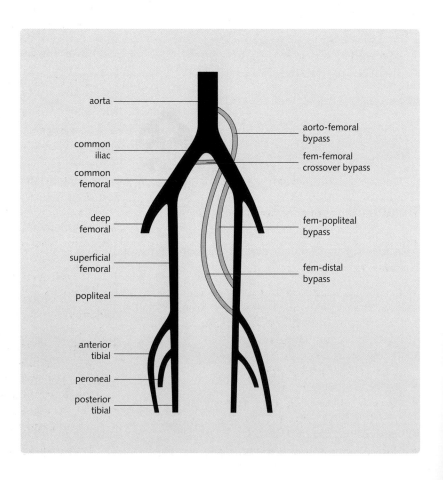

necrotic and non-viable, amputation should be performed.

Peripheral vascular disease is very common in diabetics and smokers. It is important to establish the claudication distance, i.e. how far the patient can walk before onset of pain. This helps determine whether the management should be conservative or surgical. 'Stop smoking, start walking' is a good starting point for treatment.

SHOCK AND HAEMORRHAGE

Shock

Definition

Shock is an acute failure of the cardiovascular system to adequately perfuse the tissues of the body. There are four major shock categories depending upon the causative factor:

- Hypovolaemic shock.
- Distributive shock.
- Cardiogenic shock.
- Obstructive shock.

Symptoms

The symptoms of shock are:

- Faintness, light-headedness, dizziness.
- Sweating, pallor.
- Reduced level of consciousness.

Signs

The classical signs of shock are:

- Pale, cold, clammy skin caused by cutaneous vasoconstriction in an effort to conserve blood flow to the vital organs and sweating caused by sympathetic stimulation.
- Rapid, weak pulse caused by tachycardia and decreased stroke volume.
- Reduced pulse pressure.
- Rapid, shallow breathing.
- Impaired urine output.
- Muscular weakness.
- Confusion or reduced awareness.

Hypovolaemic shock

This results from a fall in circulating blood volume caused by either:

- External fluid loss (e.g. vomiting, diarrhoea, haemorrhage).
- Internal fluid loss (e.g. pancreatitis, severe burns, internal bleeding).

Distributive shock

This is not due to a loss of fluid, but maldistribution of fluid as it leaves the intravascular compartment. The two main causes are:

- Sepsis.
- Anaphylaxis.

Septic shock

Septic shock is caused by toxins (e.g. endotoxin) released from bacteria during infection. The patient may have warm skin, but will have a low blood pressure due to inappropriate vasodilatation. Treatment is with fluid replacement, antibiotics and if severe can include noradrenaline and vasoconstrictors. Artificial ventilation is sometimes required for lung involvement if ARDS (adult respiratory distress syndrome) develops.

Anaphylactic shock

This is a type I hypersensitivity reaction, which is an immediate IgE-mediated immune response to an antigen in the body to which the patient is allergic. It leads to circulatory collapse, dyspnoea, and even death.

The IgE immune response consists of the activation of basophils and mast cells (basophils are mobile in the blood, mast cells are fixed in tissue). The degranulation of these cells leads to release of histamine and other factors. Prostaglandins, leukotrienes, thromboxane, and platelet activation factors are also synthesized and released. The results are as follows:

- Generalized peripheral vasodilatation, which leads to hypotension.
- Increased vascular permeability reducing plasma volume.
- Bronchial smooth muscle constriction, which leads to dyspnoea.
- Oral, laryngeal, and pharyngeal oedema.
- Urticaria and flushing.

Death may result from the circulatory collapse.

Treatment consists of immediate intramuscular adrenaline, anti-histamine (e.g. chlorpheniramine) and an infusion of hydrocortisone (a glucocorticoid).

An anaphylactoid reaction produces a similar picture to that described above, but it is caused by the direct effects of a substance on mast cells and basophils (i.e. it is not mediated by IgE). This sometimes occurs with radio-opaque contrast media.

> Anaphylaxis may occur with anaesthetic gases and antibiotics. The initial treatment is Airway, Breathing, Circulation. Oxygen; fluids and adrenaline should be given immediately. Steroids and antihistamines should be given shortly after. The patient should be referred to an immunologist, and carry an alert bracelet if appropriate.

Cardiogenic shock

This is caused by an interruption of cardiac function such that the heart is unable to maintain the circulation, i.e. pump failure. It usually has an acute onset, but it may be a result of worsening heart failure. Causes include:

- Myocardial infarction.
- Arrhythmia.
- Myocarditis.

Valve failure, caused by infective endocarditis or mitral valve prolapse for example, may also result in shock.

Obstructive shock

In obstructive shock there is a direct obstruction to blood leaving the heart or great vessels, for example:

- Cardiac tamponade.
- Pulmonary embolism.
- Tension pneumothorax.

Haemorrhage

A 10% blood loss produces no change in blood pressure. A 20–30% blood loss may cause shock, but it is not usually life threatening. A 30–40% blood loss produces severe or irreversible shock (50–70 mmHg fall in blood pressure). Respiratory rate is a much more sensitive indicator of blood loss than pulse rate or blood pressure, as Fig. 6.3 shows. Hypotension is an indirect result of blood loss. It is caused by a decreased blood volume, reducing venous return to the heart. A reduced end-diastolic volume reduces the strength of contraction and, therefore, stroke volume.

The body responds in different ways to rectify the loss of pressure and volume. The response is often subdivided into:

- An immediate response occurring within seconds (Fig. 6.4).
- An intermediate response occurring within minutes or hours (Fig. 6.5).
- A long-term response occurring within days or weeks (Fig. 6.6).

Treatment is to prevent further blood loss and volume expansion with intravenous fluids. Haemorrhage differs from other causes of hypovolaemia however as red cells, clotting factors and other components of plasma are also lost.

HYPERTENSION

Current World Health Organization (WHO) recommendations define hypertension as a resting blood pressure above 140 mmHg systolic and/or 90 mmHg diastolic in those under 50 years, and 160 mmHg systolic and/or 95 mmHg diastolic in older patients, although these criteria are somewhat arbitrary. Cardiovascular disease risks increase with blood pressure even within the normal range. Using the WHO criteria, up to 25% of the population may have hypertension.

Classification

Hypertension is classified according to both underlying cause and clinical progression. Primary (essential) hypertension accounts for 90% of hypertensive patients; the precise aetiology is unknown, but it is probably multifactorial. Predisposing factors include:

- Age (blood pressure rises with age).
- Obesity.
- Excessive alcohol intake.
- High salt intake.
- Genetic susceptibility.

Adaptations to acute haemorrhage

Parameter	Class I	Class II	Class III	Class IV
Blood loss (%)	0–15	15–30	30–40	>40
Blood loss (mL)	0–750	750–1500	1500–2000	>2000
Pulse rate	↔	↑	↑	↑↑
Respiratory rate	↔	↑	↑↑	↑↑
Capillary refill time	↔	↔	↑	↑↑
Blood pressure	↔	↔	Narrowing of pulse pressure	↓

Fig. 6.3 Physiological adaptations to acute haemorrhage.

Fig. 6.4 Immediate response to haemorrhage (ADH, antidiuretic hormone; BP, blood pressure; CO, cardiac output; HR, heart rate; SV, stroke volume; TPR, total peripheral resistance).

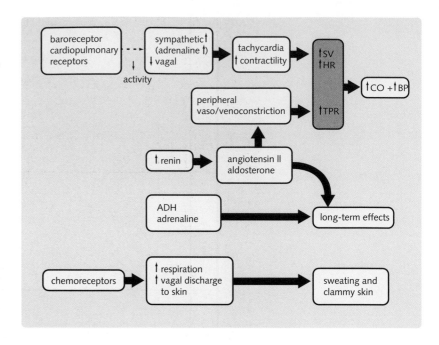

Fig. 6.5 Intermediate response to haemorrhage.

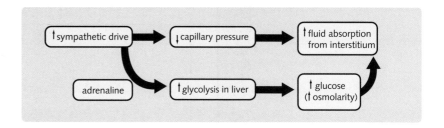

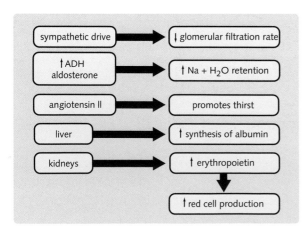

Fig. 6.6 Long-term response to haemorrhage (ADH, antidiuretic hormone).

Smoking increases cardiovascular risk in hypertensive patients. Secondary hypertension accounts for the remaining 10% of cases. Here, the hypertension arises as a result of other disease processes (see Fig. 6.7)

The clinical progression of hypertension can be classified as benign or malignant. Benign hypertension is a stable elevation of blood pressure over a period of many years (usually recognized in patients aged over 40 years). Malignant (accelerated) hypertension is an acute, severe elevation of blood pressure.

Secondary causes of hypertension				
Physiological	**Renal**	**Drugs**	**Endocrine**	**Anatomical**
Pregnancy	Renal parochymal disease Renovascular disorders Renal artery stenosis	Oral contraceptives Steroids NSAIDs	Acromegaly Cushings Conns syndrome Phaeochromocytoma Carcinoid Congenital adrenal hyperplasia	Coarctation of aorta Aortitis

Fig. 6.7 Secondary causes of hypertension (NSAIDs, non-steroidal anti-inflammatory drugs).

The distinction between primary and secondary hypertension is of great clinical significance, since only in the latter case is treatment of the underlying cause possible.

Complications

Hypertension is a major risk factor for:

- Atherosclerosis.
- Cerebrovascular disease.
- Aortic aneurysm.
- Cardiac failure (which is the cause of death in one-third of patients).
- Atrial fibrillation.
- Renal failure.
- Visual disturbance (caused by papilloedema and retinal haemorrhages).

Note that initially hypertension is usually asymptomatic, and in essential hypertension no obvious cause can be found. This can affect compliance with therapy, especially if drugs have too many side effects.

Hypertensive vascular disease

Hypertension not only accelerates atherosclerosis, but it also results in characteristic changes to arterioles and small arteries – arteriolosclerosis. All these changes are associated with narrowing of the vessel lumen. Changes in benign hypertension include:

- In arteries – muscular hypertrophy of the media, reduplication of the external lamina, and intimal thickening.
- In arterioles – hyaline arteriosclerosis (protein deposits in wall).
- In vessels of the brain – microaneurysms (Charcot–Bouchard aneurysms) can occur.

Other changes are associated with, but not restricted to, malignant hypertension. Hyperplastic arteriosclerosis, with reduplication of basement membrane and muscular hypertrophy solely within the intima, can occur in arteries and arterioles.

When these changes are associated with fibrin deposition (also known as fibrinoid changes) and necrosis of the vessel wall, the condition is known as necrotizing arteriolitis. These changes frequently affect the renal arterioles to produce nephrosclerosis, which may impair renal function or exacerbate hypertension through the renin–angiotensin system.

Hypertensive heart disease

Systemic (left-sided) hypertensive heart disease

Criteria for diagnosis of systemic hypertensive heart disease are:

- History of hypertension (>140/90 mmHg).
- Left ventricular hypertrophy (wall thickness measuring >15 mm, weight >500 g, or ECG changes).
- Absence of any other causes of hypertrophy.

In hypertensive heart disease, changes that are initially adaptive lead to cardiac dilatation, congestive heart failure, and even sudden death. The heart adapts with hypertrophy of the left ventricular wall, initially without any change in ventricular volume. Histologically this is characterized by enlargement of the myocytes and their nuclei (hypertrophy). In the long term, interstitial fibrosis and myocyte atrophy occur, causing ventricular dilatation.

Pulmonary hypertensive heart disease (cor pulmonale)

Pulmonary hypertensive heart disease can be defined as right ventricular hypertrophy (wall thickness measuring >4 mm) as a result of hypertension in the pulmonary circulation caused by a primary lung pathology.

Pulmonary hypertension can be classified as:

- Right ventricular hypertrophy and failure (also known as chronic pulmonary hypertension or cor pulmonale).
- Acute pulmonary hypertension (a sudden onset usually after a large pulmonary embolism).

Right ventricular hypertrophy and failure is a chronic disease of right ventricular pressure load (e.g. pulmonary vasoconstriction in hypoxia caused by high altitude or in chronic obstructive airways disease). Right ventricular dilatation may cause tricuspid regurgitation.

Pulmonary artery hypertension may be caused by heart disease (left ventricular failure, mitral valve disease, cardiac shunts) or lung disease (primary pulmonary hypertension, interstitial fibrosis, pulmonary emboli).

Antihypertensive drugs

Angiotensin-converting enzyme inhibitors

Angiotensin-converting enzyme (ACE) inhibitors (e.g. captopril, enalapril, perindopril) inhibit the conversion of angiotensin I to angiotensin II by ACE (Fig. 6.8). They also inhibit bradykinin (a vasodilator) breakdown by ACE. They are now becoming a first-line treatment, but they should not be used to treat patients with severe renal artery stenosis as this predisposes to flash pulmonary oedema, renal ischaemia and subsequent failure.

The side effects are:

- First-dose hypotension.
- Skin rash.
- Coughing.
- Renal impairment.

There are a number of once-a-day preparations (e.g. lisinopril and ramipril) which have a lower incidence of first-dose hypotension.

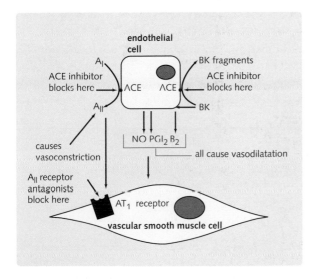

Fig. 6.8 Action of angiotensin-converting enzyme (ACE) inhibitors and angiotensin II (A$_{II}$) receptor antagonists (A$_I$, angiotensin I, A$_{II}$, angiotensin II; AT$_1$, angiotensin II receptor type 1; B$_2$, activated bradykinin-activated by endothelial cell; BK, bradykinin; NO, nitric oxide; PGI$_2$, prostacyclin).

Angiotensin II receptor antagonists

Angiotensin II receptor antagonists (e.g. losartan) inhibit the angiotensin II receptor and prevent the action of angiotensin II (Fig. 6.8). They are useful when ACE inhibitors have produced an intolerable cough (possibly caused by elevated bradykinin).

Diuretics

Usually a thiazide-type diuretic is used (e.g. bendrofluazide). These drugs inhibit sodium reabsorption in the distal renal tubule, which causes increased salt and water excretion, decreasing blood volume and decreasing blood pressure. Side effects in high doses are:

- Hypokalaemia (low K$^+$) leading to arrhythmia and muscle fatigue.
- Hyperuricaemia (high uric acid) causing gout.
- Hyperglycaemia (raised blood glucose).
- Increased low-density lipoprotein (LDL) and very low-density lipoprotein (VLDL) leading to atherosclerosis.

Other diuretics may also occasionally be used, see p. 85.

Beta-blockers

Beta-blockers are antagonists of β-adrenoceptors. They block sympathetic activity in the heart (β$_1$), peripheral vasculature (β$_2$), and other tissues including the bronchi (β$_2$).

In the heart, this results in a decrease in heart rate and myocardial contractility. Renin release from the juxtaglomerular cells is reduced and there is a central action, reducing sympathetic drive. These effects combine to lower blood pressure, but only in hypertensive patients.

The effect of β-blockers on the peripheral vasculature leads to a loss of β-mediated vasodilatation causing an unopposed α-vasoconstriction. This may initially cause an increase in vascular resistance, elevating blood pressure, but, in long-term use, the vascular resistance returns to pretreatment levels. However, peripheral blood flow may still be reduced, leading patients to complain of cold extremities.

Some β-blockers can preferentially act on β$_1$-adrenoceptors, being more cardioselective; however, even these drugs have some blocking effect on the β$_2$-adrenoceptor, and they should be given to asthmatic patients with extreme caution.

Types of β-blockers include:

- Propranolol, atenolol (act on β_1, β_2).
- Metoprolol, bisoprolol (selective β_1-blockers).

The main side effects of β-blockers are:

- Bronchoconstriction, leading to worsening asthma or chronic obstructive airways disease.
- Bradycardia.
- Hypoglycaemia.
- Fatigue and lethargy.
- Impotence.
- Sleep disturbance, nightmares, and vivid dreams (particularly propranolol).
- Rebound hypertension if stopped suddenly.

Alpha-blockers

Alpha-blockers (e.g. prazosin and doxazosin) are antagonists of α-adrenoceptors. There is postsynaptic block of α_1-adrenoceptors, which prevents sympathetic tonic drive and leads to vasodilatation. Therefore, there is a decrease in total peripheral resistance and thus a decrease in blood pressure. Doxazosin is often used for labile (catecholamine-mediated) hypertension.

Side effects of α-blockers are:

- Postural hypotension caused by loss of sympathetic vasoconstriction.
- First-dose phenomenon of rapid hypotension when initially administered.

Other sympatholytics

Adrenergic neuron blockers (e.g. guanethidine) prevent the release of noradrenaline from post-ganglionic neurons. They are rarely used now because they affect supine blood pressure control, and they may cause postural hypotension. They may be useful with other therapy in resistant hypertension.

Centrally acting α_2-agonists (e.g. methyldopa) decrease central sympathetic drive by displacing noradrenaline with a false transmitter (e.g. methylnoradrenaline from methyldopa). Release of the false transmitter is more active on α_2 pre-synaptic negative feedback receptors than on α_1, reducing transmitter release and ultimately blood pressure. They are used to treat hypertension in pregnancy because more modern drugs have never been tested in pregnancy.

Calcium antagonists

Calcium antagonists (e.g. verapamil, nifedipine, amlodipine, diltiazem) block voltage-gated calcium channels in myocardium and vascular smooth muscle. This causes a decrease in myocardial contractility, electrical conductance and vascular tone.

Calcium antagonists interfere with the action of various vasoconstrictor agonists (e.g. noradrenaline, angiotensin II, thrombin). All may precipitate heart failure (but this risk is reduced with nifedipine and nifedipine-like drugs, e.g. amlodipine).

Verapamil and diltiazem decrease heart rate by causing an inhibition of conduction through the AV node. They should be used only very cautiously with β-blockers as this may lead to heart block. The main side effect of these drugs is constipation.

Nifedipine and amlodipine relax vascular smooth muscle, dilating arteries. The main side effects are headache and ankle oedema.

Diltiazem also decreases vascular tone, hence its use as an anti-anginal. Its main side effect is bradycardia.

Potassium channel agonists

Potassium channel agonists (e.g. nicorandil) open ATP-dependent K^+ channels. Opening of K^+ channels hyperpolarizes vascular smooth muscle cells, thereby making depolarization harder to achieve. This reduces the stimulation by vasoconstricting agonists on the muscle cells.

Potassium channel agonists are used only in severe hypertension when other methods have failed (diazoxide is used in hypertensive emergencies). They are usually used with a β-blocker and thiazide diuretic to counteract side effects.

Side effects of potassium channel agonists are:

- Increased hair growth (with minoxidil).
- Salt and water retention, leading to oedema (use thiazide).
- Reflex sympathetic activation causing tachycardia (use β-blocker).

Combinations

ACE inhibitors are being used increasingly as a first-line treatment for hypertension as they carry a reduced risk of side effects. They can be combined with thiazide treatment, but caution should be used with existing diuretic treatment due to the risk of a collapse in blood pressure in volume depleted patients. β-Blockers have traditionally been used with a thiazide if a thiazide has not been effective alone.

After these options have failed or are contraindicated, calcium antagonists should be tried. Diuretics may be used in addition, but verapamil should not be combined with β-blockers.

In severe hypertension where the above therapies have been tried or are contraindicated, then the vasodilators, α-blockers, and centrally acting drugs may be used. They may be used in conjunction with an ACE inhibitor, or a thiazide and a β-blocker, although doxazosin is being used more frequently in preference to diuretics and β-blockers because of its vasodilator effect and minimal side effects.

LIPIDS AND THE CARDIOVASCULAR SYSTEM

Lipid transport and metabolism

The insolubility of lipids in plasma means a special transport mechanism is required. This is provided by lipid–protein complexes known as lipoproteins, while the individual proteins are known as apolipoproteins. The apolipoproteins also act as receptors for cell surface proteins, which determine the destination of different lipoproteins. Low-density lipoprotein (LDL) is the main lipoprotein involved in the transport of cholesterol. Fig. 6.9 shows the main transport pathways for lipids from the diet (exogenous) and for lipids from the body's stores (endogenous).

It is thought that lipoprotein A is a prothrombotic lipoprotein that is particularly involved in coronary disease, while high levels of high-density lipoprotein (HDL) are protective. The classification of lipoproteins is outlined in Fig. 6.10.

Hyperlipidaemia

Hyperlipidaemia (Fig. 6.11) can be classified as hypertriglyceridaemia (raised triglycerides – also called triacylglycerides), hypercholesterolaemia (raised cholesterol), or hyperlipoproteinaemia (raised lipoproteins).

Effects of hyperlipidaemia
Atherosclerosis

There is a strong correlation between cholesterol levels and death rates from ischaemic vascular disease. There is an even stronger correlation between fibrinogen levels and ischaemic vascular disease. It must, therefore, be remembered that atherosclerosis is a multifactorial disease.

It is thought that LDL damages the arterial wall by producing oxygen radicals, or exacerbates wall injury from other causes. Atheromatous plaques may develop in this damaged arterial wall. HDL however is protective against atherosclerosis.

Acute pancreatitis

Acute pancreatitis can result from hypertriglyceridaemia.

Subcutaneous deposits

Subcutaneous deposits of lipids are often painful, and can be found in the skin usually around the eyes (xanthelasma) and in tendons (tendon xanthomas). They are usually diagnostic of hyperlipidaemia.

Treatment of hyperlipidaemia

Hyperlipidaemia can be treated by diet or drugs.

Dietary treatment involves reduction of calorific intake, saturated fats, cholesterol, and alcohol; supplements of omega-3 fats (present in fish oils) are given, increasing HDL levels, which is beneficial.

Indications for drug therapy are:

- High LDL levels, which must be treated if arterial disease is present.
- High triglycerides, which need to be treated only if symptomatic (e.g. causing xanthomas or pancreatitis).
- Low HDL levels.

Drugs used to lower cholesterol

Statins (e.g. simvastatin, atorvastatin)
Statins are β-hydroxy-β-methylglutaryl coenzyme A (HMG CoA) reductase inhibitors. The liver compensates for the decreased cholesterol synthesis by increasing LDL receptors, which decreases plasma levels of LDL-cholesterol. They are used to treat most hypercholesterolaemias, and they are very

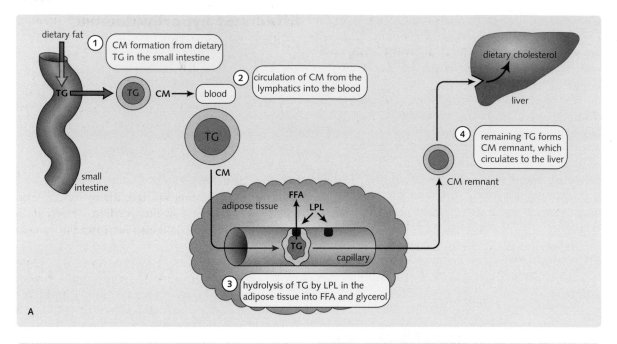

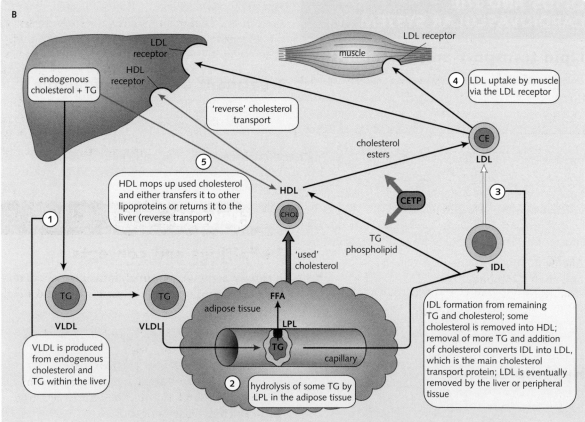

Fig. 6.9 (A) Exogenous and (B) endogenous lipid transport pathways (CE, cholesterol esters; CETP, cholesterol ester transfer protein; CM, chylomicron; FFA, free fatty acid; HDL, high-density lipoprotein; IDL, intermediate-density lipoprotein; LDL, low-density lipoprotein; LPL, lipoprotein lipase; TG, triacylglycerol; VLDL, very low-density lipoprotein).

Classification of lipoproteins		
Particle	Source	Predominantly transports
Chylomicron (CM)	Gut	Triacylglycerol
Very low-density lipoprotein (VLDL)	Liver	Triacylglycerol
Intermediate-density lipoprotein (IDL)	Catabolism	Cholesterol
Low-density lipoprotein (LDL)	Catabolism	Cholesterol
High-density lipoprotein (HDL)	Catabolism	Cholesterol
Lipoprotein A	Liver, gut	—

Fig. 6.10 Classification of lipoproteins.

be used alone, or in combination with a statin to further lower cholesterol.

Probucol
Probucol causes a 10% reduction in LDL-cholesterol, but it also lowers HDL and remains in the body for months. It has some antioxidant activity, which may reduce atherosclerosis formation.

Drugs used to lower triglyceride levels

Nicotinic acid
Nicotinic acid inhibits VLDL synthesis by the liver, leading to a decrease in intermediate density lipoprotein (IDL) and LDL. It also increases lipoprotein lipase (LPL) activity.

Nicotinic acid can be used for most types of hyperlipidaemia, usually in conjunction with a resin (see above). Its main side effects are rashes, nausea, abnormal liver function, and a prostaglandin-mediated cutaneous reaction.

Fibrates
Gemfibrozil reduces lipolysis of triglycerides in adipose tissue, leading to decreased hepatic production of VLDL. Bezafibrate increases LPL activity, which leads to decreased VLDL and decreased triglycerides, but it may increase LDL.

Fibrates are used mainly in familial hyperlipidaemia. Gemfibrozil is the better drug as it does not increase LDL. The main side effects include nausea, abdominal discomfort and flu-like symptoms.

effective if used in conjunction with a resin (up to 50% reduction in cholesterol levels). They are currently the only lipid-lowering treatment for which there is good evidence for reduced mortality.

The main side effects include reversible myositis and disturbed liver function tests.

Hyperlipidaemias must be remembered as controllable causes of coronary heart disease, especially in young adults.

Bile acid binding resins (e.g. colestipol and cholestyramine)
Colestipol and cholestyramine inhibit reabsorption of cholesterol in the gut. They bind to bile salts in the gut and stop their reabsorption. This leads to increased excretion and decreased absorption of cholesterol. To compensate, the liver increases cholesterol conversion into bile salts and also increases LDL receptors. This removes LDL-cholesterol from circulation. They can aggravate hypertriglyceridaemia.

Ezetimibe
This is a novel, orally acting selective inhibitor of dietary and biliary absorption of cholesterol. It may

ANEURYSMS

Definitions and concepts

An aneurysm is an abnormal, focal, permanent dilatation of an artery or part of the heart (Fig. 6.12). It is caused by a weakening of the wall:

- A true aneurysm is surrounded by all three layers of the arterial wall.
- A false aneurysm occurs when there is an actual hole in all or part of the arterial wall, which causes blood to move extravascularly, producing a haematoma.
- A dissecting aneurysm occurs when the blood is contained between the internal layers of the arterial wall and progresses by splitting the muscular layers (Fig. 6.13).

Classification of hyperlipidaemias					
Condition	Elevated lipoprotein	Elevated lipid	Biochemical defect	Drug therapy	Prevalence
Single gene defect					
Familial lipoprotein lipase (LPL) deficiency (type I)	CMs	Triacylglyceride	Low or absent LPL activity	Diet alone	Rare
Familial hypercholesterolaemia (type IIa)	LDL	Cholesterol	Deficiency of LDL receptors (none in homozygotes)	Statin, resin	Common
Familial combined hyperlipidaemia (type IIb)	VLDL, LDL	Triacylglyceride, cholesterol	Overproduction of apo-B	Fibrate	Common
Familial hyperlipoproteinaemia (type III)	CM remnants, IDL	Triacylglyceride, cholesterol	Abnormal apo-E	Fibrate	Rare
Familial hypertriglyceridaemia (type IV)	VLDL	Triacylglyceride	Overproduction of VLDL by the liver	Fibrate	Common
Familial hypertriglyceridaemia (type V)	VLDL, CMs	Triacylglyceride, cholesterol	Overproduction of VLDL by the liver	Fibrate	Rare
Multifactorial					
Hypertriglyceridaemia	VLDL	Triacylglyceride	Unknown	Fibrate	Common
Hypercholesterolaemia	LDL	Cholesterol	Unknown	Statin, resin	Common

Fig. 6.11 Classification of hyperlipidaemias. Familial, heritable abnormalities of lipid metabolism are classified according to Fredrickson type (types I–V) on the underlying genetic mutations. Hyperlipidaemia may also be multifactorial or idiopathic, without a currently identified or discrete genetic basis. These are clinically the most common in older patients. (CM, chylomicron; IDL, intermediate-density lipoprotein; LDL, low-density lipoprotein; VLDL, very low-density lipoprotein.)

Aneurysms are caused by:

- Atherosclerosis. Plaque formation causes medial destruction and wall thinning. This commonly occurs in the abdominal aorta.
- Cystic medial degeneration – mucinous degeneration of the media with fragmentation of the elastic tissue. This is often seen in dissecting aortic aneurysms.
- Syphilis.
- Trauma.
- Vasculitides (especially polyarteritis nodosa).
- Congenital defects (e.g. berry aneurysms).
- Infections (mycotic aneurysms).

Aneurysms are often described by their shape. They are either fusiform (spindle shaped, being tapered at either end) or saccular (sac-like).

Mycotic aneurysms are aneurysms caused by infection. Bacteria within septic emboli that lodge in arteries may cause destruction of the arterial wall.

Turbulence of blood within an aneurysm frequently leads to the formation of a thrombus, increasing the risk of rupture.

Abdominal aortic aneurysm

The prevalence of abdominal aortic aneurysms is 3% in men aged over 50 years.

The aneurysm is usually found proximal to the iliac bifurcation of the abdominal aorta. The patient may be asymptomatic or have abdominal/back pain if there is compression of retroperitoneal structures.

Leaking and rupture with resultant haemorrhage is the most serious complication; the patient may present acutely shocked. Fistulae into the gut or vena cava may rarely occur.

Hypertension increases the risk of rupture, which occurs in approximately 30% of patients. The risk of rupture increases with the size of the aneurysm, hence all those >5 cm are considered suitable for surgery.

Surgery aims to prevent rupture. Elective surgery has an operative mortality of 5%, rising to 50% if the aneurysm ruptures. Treatment aims to replace the aneurysm with a synthetic graft, and is increasingly performed as an endovascular procedure in contrast to the conventional open repair.

Postoperative complications include myocardial infarction and renal failure.

> Abdominal aortic aneurysm is very common, especially in hypertensive male smokers. Treatment is initially conservative by monitoring of the aneurysm with ultrasound. Surgery, either open or endovascular repair, should only be considered when the risk of the aneurysm rupturing exceeds the risks of surgery. This is thought to be at a size >5 cm.

Syphilitic (luetic) aneurysm

Syphilitic (luetic) aneurysms can occur in the thoracic aorta of patients with tertiary syphilis.

There is inflammation of the adventitia, especially the vasa vasorum (endarteritis). This causes ischaemia and loss of muscle and elastic tissue, which leads to weakening of the arterial wall.

Microscopically the vasa vasorum have thickened walls, and they are surrounded by inflammatory cells. The aneurysm may extend backwards along the aorta to the aortic valve leading to valve regurgitation.

Fig. 6.12 Types of aneurysm: saccular, fusiform, and false.

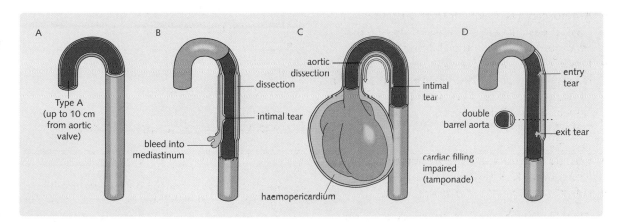

Fig. 6.13 Dissecting aortic aneurysm. (A) Type A and B dissections. Type A are within 10 cm of the aortic value; type B are beyond this. (B) Rupture into the mediastinum. (C) Rupture into the pericardium. (D) Rupture into the aorta.

Sequelae include syphilitic heart disease, compression of adjacent structures, and rupture.

Aortic dissection

In this condition, blood in the aorta is dissected into two flows: one in the normal lumen and another in one of the layers of the media (Fig. 6.13). There are two main types:

- Stanford type A involves an intimal tear in the ascending aorta within 10 cm of the aortic valve. This aneurysm can be treated by surgical replacement of the aortic arch.
- Stanford type B involves the descending thoracic aorta. As surgery here is more complex, management is medical with careful reduction in blood pressure.

Aortic dissection is seen predominantly in men aged 40–60 years with systemic hypertension, particularly in Marfan syndrome where cystic medial degeneration occurs. It may also occur as a result of trauma, especially iatrogenic (e.g. during arterial cannulation).

Clinical features include sudden onset of severe chest pain radiating to the back and downwards.

Sequelae of dissection include:

- Rupture into the thorax or abdomen.
- Occlusion of aortic branches, especially coronary, cerebral, and renal arteries.
- Extension along the aorta to include other arteries or disruption of the aortic valve.
- Cardiac tamponade caused by proximal extension and subsequent haemopericardium.

Other causes of aneurysms

Congenital causes

Berry aneurysms in the circle of Willis can be caused by focal weakness in the arterial wall of the cerebral vessels. In contrast to aortic aneurysms, they are saccular. Rupture of these occasionally occurs leading to subarachnoid haemorrhage.

Vasculitides

Two forms of vasculitis may cause aneurysm (see p. 119):

- Polyarteritis nodosa – aneurysms may form in any organ with vessels affected by the disease.

- Kawasaki syndrome – dilatation of the coronary arteries associated with arteritis is a complication of the disease.

Myocardial ischaemia

Myocardial ischaemia may lead to dilatation and aneurysm of the ventricle, which may later rupture. A similar aneurysm may also occur in Chagas' disease (trypanosomiasis).

INFLAMMATORY VASCULAR DISEASE

Concepts and classification

The vasculitides are a group of conditions characterized by vasculitis (inflammation and damage of the vessel walls), categorized in Fig. 6.14. They may be classified by pathogenesis (infective, immune-mediated, or idiopathic) or by the size of the vessel affected (large, medium, or small).

Most systemic vasculitides probably involve an immunological process. Many different processes have been described. There may be deposition of circulating antigen–antibody complexes in conditions such as systemic lupus erythematosus. Antibodies may react with fixed tissue antigens as in Kawasaki syndrome. Temporal arteritis involves delayed-type hypersensitivity reactions with granuloma formation.

Vessels affected by vasculitides		
Vessel size	Arteries	Disease
Large/ medium	Aorta Carotid Temporal	Giant cell arteritis, Takayasu's arteritis
Medium/ small	Coronary Mesenteric	Polyarteritis nodosa, Kawasaki disease
Small/ arteriole	Glomeruli and arterioles	Wegener's granulomatosis, microscopic polyarteritis nodosa
Arteriole/ capillary	—	Henoch–Schönlein purpura, cutaneous leucocytoclastic
Veins	—	Buerger's disease

Fig. 6.14 Vessels affected by vasculitides.

The presence of anti-neutrophilic cytoplasmic autoantibodies (ANCA), which react with antigens in the cytoplasm of neutrophils, can be seen in many vasculitides. The antigen may be perinuclear (p-ANCA) or cytoplasmic (c-ANCA).

Infectious vasculitides

The causes of infectious vasculitides may be:

- Bacterial (e.g. Neisseria).
- Viral (e.g. herpes).
- Other infectious causes such as Rickettsia (Rocky Mountain spotted fever), spirochaetes (syphilis), or fungi (Aspergillus).

Immunological vasculitides

The immunological vasculitides can be classified as:

- Immune complex – Henoch–Schönlein purpura, systemic lupus erythematosus.
- Direct antibody – Goodpasture's syndrome (anti-basement membrane antibodies), Kawasaki disease.
- ANCA associated – Wegener's granulomatosis, microscopic polyarteritis.
- Cell mediated – organ rejection.

Idiopathic vasculitides

Giant-cell (temporal) arteritis

Giant-cell arteritis is the most common of the vasculitides, occurring in the elderly and being rare in those younger than 55 years of age. There is focal granulomatous inflammation of medium and small arteries, especially the cranial vessels. It usually presents with headache and facial pain, or polymyalgia rheumatica (flu-like aches and fever). The erythrocyte sedimentation rate (ESR) and/or C reactive protein (CRP) are usually raised. Visual disturbances develop in about half affected individuals and may lead to blindness without prompt intervention. Diagnosis is by temporal artery biopsy; microscopically, the following signs are seen:

- Granulations with giant cells.
- General leucocytic infiltrate.
- Fibrosis of the intima and stenosis.

There is often associated thrombosis. Diagnosis is by biopsy, which may be negative in one-third of cases. Treatment is with high doses of corticosteroids.

> Giant cell arteritis commonly affects the temporal arteries and is important as it is an easily preventable cause of blindness.

Takayasu's disease (aortic arch syndrome)

Takayasu's disease typically affects females in the 20–40-year-old age group. It is most common in Asia. It is a granulomatous vasculitis of medium-to-large arteries, especially the aorta and the great vessels. Patients present with visual disturbances, neurological deficits, and diminished upper pulses ('pulseless disease'). If the renal arteries are involved, hypertension may result. There is thickening of the aortic wall with mononuclear cell infiltrates. Fibrosis and granulomas may result.

Polyarteritis nodosa

Polyarteritis nodosa is twice as common in males as in females, usually occurring in the middle aged. It is associated with the hepatitis B surface (s) antigen. p-ANCA is usually elevated.

Fibrinoid necrosis of medium-to-small arteries occurs, especially of the main viscera (e.g. coronary, renal and hepatic arteries). The pulmonary arteries are not usually affected. Presenting features can be general (e.g. fever) or relate to the specific system involved:

- Renal – hypertension, renal failure.
- Cardiac – myocardial infarction, heart failure.
- Central nervous system – hemiplegia, psychoses.
- Gastrointestinal – abdominal pain, melaena.

Segmental lesions occur, with fibrinoid necrosis of the wall and a neutrophil infiltrate. Healing results in thickening and often aneurysmal dilatation. A type of polyarteritis nodosa known as Churg–Strauss is an eosinophilic syndrome which affects the lungs. Diagnosis is by biopsy; treatment is with anti-viral therapy for hepatitis B associated polyarteritis or immunosuppression.

Kawasaki syndrome (mucocutaneous lymph node syndrome)

Kawasaki syndrome is an acute febrile illness of young children. Patients present with lymphadenopathy, rash, erythema, peeling skin, and (in 20% of those affected) coronary arteritis with aneurysms, which may lead to myocardial infarction or sudden cardiac death.

Similar lesions occur to those seen in polyarteritis nodosa. Aspirin and γ-globulin therapy is thought to prevent cardiac complications.

Microscopic polyarteritis (leucocytoclastic angiitis)

Microscopic polyarteritis is a fibrinoid necrosis of the smallest vessels, and it is thought to be a form of hypersensitivity reaction. Typically, there is an acute onset with a precipitating agent (e.g. bacteria) and involvement of the skin or viscera. There may be little neutrophilic infiltrate.

Wegener's granulomatosis

The majority of cases are in patients aged over 50 years. The condition consists of a triad of symptoms:

- Necrotizing vasculitis of the lung and upper respiratory tract.
- Granulomas of the respiratory tract.
- Glomerulonephritis of the kidneys.

c-ANCA type autoantibodies are usually present. Lesions are similar to those of polyarteritis nodosa, but granulomas also occur. Treatment is by immunosuppression (using prednisolone and cyclophosphamide).

Thromboangiitis obliterans (Buerger's disease)

Thromboangiitis obliterans is typically found in male smokers aged less than 35 years. It is twice as common in Jews as in non-Jews. It involves inflammation of the vessels of the lower limbs. Nodular phlebitis (inflammation of veins) and ischaemia of the extremities results. There is neutrophilic infiltration with thrombi and giant-cell formation.

Frequently, the condition is painful and leads to gangrene if smoking is not stopped.

Vasculitis in systemic disease

Many diseases have vasculitis as a component.

Systemic lupus erythematosus

Systemic lupus erythematosus (SLE) affects capillaries, arterioles, and venules. An inflammatory vasculitis is predominant; neutrophils are more common than lymphocytes. Vasculitic lesions on the skin, muscle, and brain are common. Raynaud's phenomenon may also be present. A similar pathology exists in other connective tissue disorders (e.g. scleroderma, cryoglobulinaemia).

Henoch–Schönlein purpura

This is a hypersensitivity reaction that is often preceded by infection. Purpuric rashes caused by inflammation of capillaries and venules are present on the legs and buttocks. Abdominal pain, arthritis, haematuria, and nephritis may also occur.

Rheumatoid vasculitis

Vasculitis is one of the extra-articular features of rheumatoid arthritis.

Infectious vasculitis

Systemic infections can result in a vasculitis. These often produce a purpuric rash due to a hypersensitivity reaction.

Raynaud's disease

Raynaud's disease is not strictly a vasculitis, but it is worth considering here as it has some features in common with those of other vasculitides.

Primary Raynaud's disease affects 5% of the population, and it is mainly found in young healthy women. There is pallor and cyanosis caused by vasospasm of the small arteries/arterioles in the hands and feet. The exact aetiology is unknown, but it is thought to be due to increased vasomotor responses to cold or emotion.

Secondary Raynaud's phenomenon refers to the decrease in blood flow that occurs secondary to the narrowing of the arteries that supply the extremities. It implies a known aetiology; this can be atherosclerosis, systemic lupus erythematosus, scleroderma, or Buerger's disease.

CONGENITAL ABNORMALITIES OF THE VESSELS

Vascular anatomy is complex, and it undergoes considerable remodelling during embryological development. There are many areas where alterations from the usual development can occur. These do not necessarily produce deficiencies in the flow of blood; rather, most represent an alternative supply and drainage of the same tissue. For example, errors in the remodelling of the great vessels may give rise to double inferior and superior venae cavae; this is caused by a failure of regression of a primitive element.

A vascular ring may form around the oesophagus and trachea, causing difficulty in swallowing and breathing. This is caused by a persistent right dorsal aorta or it may result from other problems in aortic arch development.

Primary lymphoedema may result from hypoplasia of the lymphatic system.

Abnormalities in the coronary circulation may sometimes be normal (e.g. when branches of the left coronary artery arise directly from the aorta), or they may lead to ischaemia and infarction of the myocardium.

Some abnormalities may even be protective. For example, sometimes the kidney has a double renal arterial supply, protecting it from under-perfusion in hypovolaemia.

Two important anomalies of the circulation are:

- Arteriovenous fistulae.
- Berry aneurysms.

Arteriovenous fistula

An arteriovenous fistula is an abnormal communication between an artery and a vein. This may be congenital in origin or secondary to trauma, inflammation, or a healed ruptured aneurysm. Fistulae may cause shunting of blood, bypassing circulations and increasing venous return, thereby increasing cardiac output. This may predispose to heart failure.

Fistulae may be seen in Paget's disease of the bone, where the increased blood flow through the affected bones may eventually lead to heart failure.

Arteriovenous fistulae are used in haemodialysis for renal patients. Artificial arteriovenous fistulae can be surgically placed between the radial artery and cephalic vein (Fig 6.15). This causes the vein to distend and thicken, enabling large bore needles to be inserted. These take blood to and from the dialysis machine.

Berry aneurysm

Berry aneurysms are found in about 2% of post mortem examinations, and they are the most common intracranial aneurysm. They are small saccular aneurysms in the cerebral vessels. They can measure about 0.2–3.0 cm in diameter, but are usually around 1.0 cm. They frequently occur at branch points in the circle of Willis (Fig. 6.16). These aneurysms are commonly seen in patients with coarctation of the aorta and polycystic renal disease.

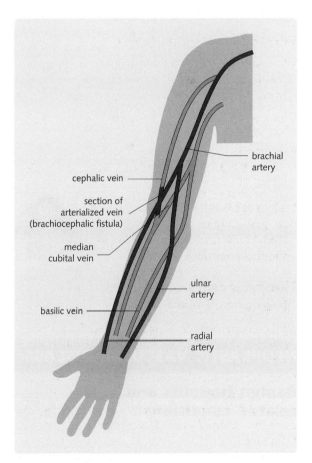

Fig. 6.15 Surgically created arteriovenous fistula.

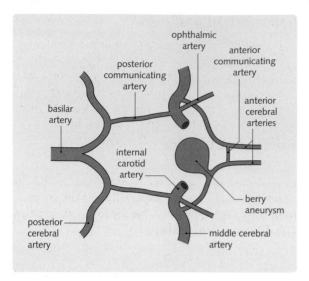

Fig. 6.16 Berry aneurysm in the circle of Willis.

Berry aneurysms are asymptomatic until they rupture (usually when the patient is aged between 40 and 60 years). Rupture is more common in males. Predisposing factors to rupture include smoking, hypertension, and atheroma. The original outpouching is caused by local focal wall weakness. This then gets larger as a result of the haemodynamics in the lumen. Eventually rupture may occur. Rupture of berry aneurysms results in a subarachnoid haemorrhage, presenting with a sudden-onset severe headache which may be fatal.

Berry aneurysms are common and can be corrected surgically, so it is important to remember this as a cause of acute severe headache.

NEOPLASTIC VASCULAR DISEASE

Benign tumours and related conditions

Haemangioma

Haemangiomas are common, especially in children; they make up approximately 7% of all benign tumours. Haemangiomas are usually subdivided into capillary haemangioma, juvenile capillary haemangioma, cavernous haemangioma and granuloma pyogenicum.

Capillary haemangioma

Capillary haemangiomas occur mostly in skin and mucous membranes. These are well-defined, encapsulated aggregates of capillaries. They may be thrombosed.

Juvenile capillary ('strawberry') haemangioma

Juvenile capillary haemangiomas are present at birth on the face and scalp of infants. They grow rapidly for the first few months then regress and disappear by the age of 5 years.

Cavernous haemangioma

Cavernous haemangiomas are large, cavernous, vascular channels that are not encapsulated. They involve skin, mucous membranes, the central nervous system, and the liver.

Granuloma pyogenicum

Granuloma pyogenicum is an ulcerated version of capillary haemangioma, often caused by trauma. Typically, it is composed of capillaries with oedema, inflammatory cells, and granulation tissue. Granuloma gravidum occurs in the gum of up to 5% of pregnant women.

Glomangioma

Glomangiomas are painful tumours of the glomus body (a receptor in the smooth muscle of arteries that is sensitive to temperature; i.e. at arteriovenous anastomoses in the skin). Glomangiomas are usually found in fingers or nail beds. They are branching vascular channels with aggregates of glomus bodies.

Telangiectasia

Telangiectasias are aggregations of prominent small vessels in the skin or mucous membranes. They are probably not a true neoplasm, but are either congenital or an exaggeration of existing vessels.

Naevus flammeus (ordinary birthmark)

Naevus flammeus is a macular lesion with vessel dilatation. Most regress, except the 'port-wine stain' naevi, which persist and are a sign of the Sturge–Weber syndrome (neurocutaneous angiomas).

Spider naevi

Spider naevi are minute, often pulsatile arterioles occurring around a central core, usually above the waist. They are associated with hyperoestrogen states (e.g. cirrhosis and pregnancy).

Osler–Weber–Rendu disease (hereditary haemorrhagic telangiectasia)

This disease is a rare autosomal dominant condition, characterized by multiple, small aneurysms on the skin and mucous membranes. Patients present with bleeding usually from the nose, mouth or rectum.

Bacillary angiomatosis

Bacillary angiomatosis is a fatal disease caused by Rickettsia-like bacteria. There is proliferation of blood vessels in the skin, lymph nodes, and organs of immunocompromised patients. Treatment with erythromycin is curative.

Intermediate-grade tumours

Haemangioendothelioma

Haemangioendotheliomas are neoplasms that show both benign and malignant characteristics (i.e. some are benign, others are malignant). They consist of vascular channels with masses of spindle-shaped plump cells of endothelial origin.

Malignant tumours

Angiosarcoma (haemangiosarcoma)

Angiosarcomas are rare, but very aggressive tumours that metastasize widely. They are found in skin, breast, liver, and spleen, especially in the elderly. There are small, discrete, red nodules that change into large, white masses, in which cells of all differentiations are found.

Haemangiopericytoma

Haemangiopericytoma is a malignant tumour of pericytes occurring in the lower extremities or in the retroperitoneum. About half of all these tumours metastasize.

Kaposi's sarcoma

Kaposi's sarcoma is a malignant tumour of unknown origin, but probably from lymphatic endothelium. Purple papules/plaques are found in the skin, mucosa, or viscera. Microscopically, it is composed of sheets of spindle-shaped plump cells with intermingled red blood cells and vascular channels.

There are four types of this disease:

Classic Kaposi's sarcoma
Classic Kaposi's sarcoma affects mainly elderly Eastern European men, especially Ashkenazi Jews. Multiple red plaques occur on the lower extremities. The disease is rarely fatal.

African Kaposi's sarcoma
African Kaposi's sarcoma affects mainly younger men in equatorial Africa. Clinically, it is similar to classic Kaposi's sarcoma.

Transplant-associated Kaposi's sarcoma
Transplant-associated Kaposi's sarcoma occurs in immunosuppressed patients. It involves the skin and viscera. Lesions regress when immunosuppression is stopped.

HIV-associated Kaposi's sarcoma
HIV-associated Kaposi's sarcoma may occur in the skin, mucous membranes, lymph nodes, viscera, or gastrointestinal tract. This is an AIDS-defining illness, and it often responds to cytotoxic drugs or α-interferon.

DISEASES OF THE VEINS AND LYMPHATICS

Varicose veins

Varicose veins are tortuous, distended superficial veins, usually of the lower limbs, caused by a persistent increased intraluminal pressure. They occur in 10–20% of the normal population, with women being more affected than men. Risk factors include:

- Pregnancy.
- Obesity.
- Prolonged standing.
- Previous deep vein thrombosis.
- Familial tendency.
- Tumours compressing the deep veins.

Aetiology

There are superficial and deep veins in the lower limb, which are interconnected by perforating veins (Fig. 6.17). Blood is returned mainly through the deep veins to the thoracic compartment by the skeletal pumping effect of the calf muscles. If there is a blockage of the deep veins (e.g. by thrombosis) or there are faulty valves in the perforating veins, then blood will move from the deep veins into the superficial veins. This will lead to distension and further valvular incompetence, resulting in stasis of blood. Oedema and changes in the skin take place (e.g. ulceration, see p. 161) which fail to heal because there is an impaired circulation.

Histologically, the venous walls will become thin where there is dilatation. Thrombosis may be seen in the superficial vein walls, but this rarely causes emboli.

Sequelae

Sequelae of varicose veins include:

- Varicose ulcers.
- Dermatitis.
- Thromboemboli.

Varicose veins do not always require treatment. Occasionally, patients complain of a dragging sensation, bleeding or are disturbed by the appearance of their legs. In these patients, surgery may be appropriate to remove the distended veins. Recurrence is a significant risk.

> Varicose veins affect a large number of people, those who stand for long periods of time, e.g. teachers, being particularly at risk. Treatment may be conservative, i.e. compression bandaging, or surgical. Surgical treatment may be local, e.g. injection of sclerosant into the dilated vein, or generalized, e.g. tying off the incompetent valve and stripping out the dilated vein.

Fig. 6.17 Perforating veins of the lower limbs.

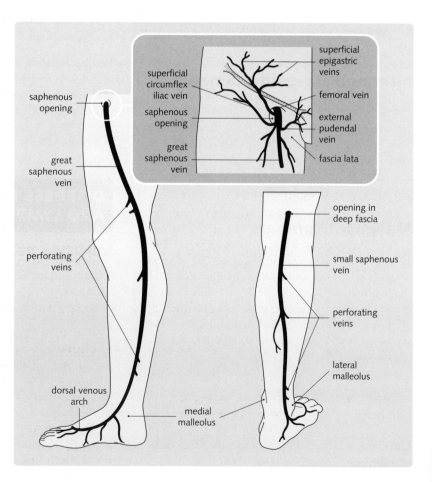

Other sites of varicosities

These are as follows:

- Haemorrhoids (piles) are distended submucosal veins in the anal canal that may protrude through the anus. Bleeding and pain may result from trauma, protrusion, or spasm of the anal sphincter.
- Varicocoele is a distension of the veins of the pampiniform plexus in the spermatic cord.
- Oesophageal varices are distended veins at the oesophageal–gastric junction. They are caused by portal hypertension, usually as a result of liver cirrhosis.

Deep vein thrombosis and thrombophlebitis

Thrombosis within a vein is termed phlebothrombosis – the term 'deep vein thrombosis' is more specific. Phlebothrombosis usually causes inflammation in the wall of the vein, which is then termed thrombophlebitis. Risk factors for thrombosis are used to formulate a Well's score (Fig 6.18).

Thrombosis mainly affects the following:

- Deep leg veins (90% of thromboses; most commonly in the thigh). Commonly they throw off emboli that impact in the pulmonary circulation.
- Periprostatic plexus in men.
- Ovarian and pelvic veins in women.

Clinical features of thrombosis vary:

- It may be asymptomatic.
- It may present with pulmonary emboli (hypoxia, chest pain, dyspnoea or collapse).
- It may cause calf pain, with swelling, redness, and distended superficial veins. The affected calf is warmer, and there may be ankle oedema.
- If severe, occlusion may lead to cyanosis of the limb, severe oedema, and gangrene.

Investigation is with Doppler ultrasonography or venography. D-dimers (fibrin degradation products) may be non-specifically raised. Initial treatment is anticoagulation with heparin. The patient is mobilized and advised to wear support stockings.

In late pregnancy, phlegmasia alba dolens (painful white 'milk leg') may occur because of thrombosis of the iliofemoral veins.

Thrombophlebitis migrans (Trousseau's syndrome) refers to multiple thrombi occurring in one place and then vanishing only to occur somewhere else. It is caused by hypercoagulability states associated with malignancy (usually adenocarcinoma of the pancreas).

Lymphangitis

Lymphangitis is inflammation of the lymphatic vessels. It is frequently found in lymphatic vessels that drain a source of infection. It often presents as a cluster of red painful streaks in the skin close to an infected site. Lymphangitis very often occurs as a result of bacterial infections (especially streptococcal). If untreated with antibiotics, it may progress to involve the lymph nodes (lymphadenitis), and it may eventually lead to septicaemia.

Histologically, the wall of the lymph vessels is infiltrated by inflammatory cells. This may spread to involve surrounding structures leading to cellulitis or an abscess.

Lymphoedema

Lymphoedema is an accumulation of interstitial fluid caused by obstruction of the draining lymphatics. The oedema is usually non-pitting (pitting oedema being suggestive of hypoproteinaemia and cardiac failure). Primary lymphoedema is a result of agenesis of the lymphatic system. Secondary lymphoedema may be caused by:

- Recurrent cellulitis.
- Malignancy.
- Surgical resection of lymph nodes.
- Radiotherapy causing fibrosis.
- Filariasis – nematode worm infection that leads to elephantiasis (gross enlargement of the skin and connective tissue).
- Post-inflammatory thrombosis leading to scarring.
- Congenital abnormal lymphatics.

If lymphoedema is prolonged, fibrosis of the interstitium occurs, leading to skin thickening and permanent oedema. The skin appears to take on an orange-peel appearance (peau d'orange). Associated ulcers and brawny hardening of the skin may also take place.

If the dilated obstructed lymphatics rupture, then chyle (lymph with digested fats) may accumulate in parts of the body cavity. Chylous ascites,

Well's risk factors for DVT	
Criteria	Score
• Lower limb trauma, surgery, or immobilization in a plaster cast	+1
• Bedridden for more than three days or surgery within last four weeks	+1
• Tenderness along line of femoral or popliteal veins	+1
• Entire limb swollen	+1
• Calf more than 3cm greater in circumference, measured 10 cm below tibial tuberosity	+1
• Pitting oedema	+1
• Dilated collateral superficial veins	+1
• Past history of DVT (confirmed)	+1
• Malignancy	+1
• Intravenous drug use	+3
• Alternative diagnosis more likely than DVT	−2
DVT 'likely' if Well's >1 DVT 'unlikely' if Well's <2	

Fig. 6.18 Well's score showing risk factors for deep venous thrombosis (DVT).

chylothorax, and chylopericardium refer to the accumulation of chyle in the abdomen, thorax, and pericardium, respectively.

Neoplasms of the lymphatics

Lymphangioma

Lymphangiomas are benign tumours of the lymphatic capillaries. They are analogous to haemangiomas. There are two types: simple and cavernous.

Simple lymphangioma

Typically, a simple lymphangioma occurs on the head, neck, or axilla. It can also occur on the trunk and in viscera.

Simple lymphangiomas are cutaneous or pedunculated nodules made up of endothelium-lined spaces in a network. No blood cells are present.

Cavernous lymphangioma (cystic hygroma)

Cavernous masses are usually present in the neck or axilla in children. They are not encapsulated and they are poorly defined – and so are difficult to resect. Cavernous lymphangiomas tend to recur. There are dilated cystic spaces lined by endothelium.

Lymphangiosarcoma

Lymphangiosarcoma is a rare malignant tumour of the lymphatics with a poor prognosis. Prolonged lymphoedema is usually associated with the condition.

The tumour comprises multiple confluent nodules of vascular channels lined with endothelium.

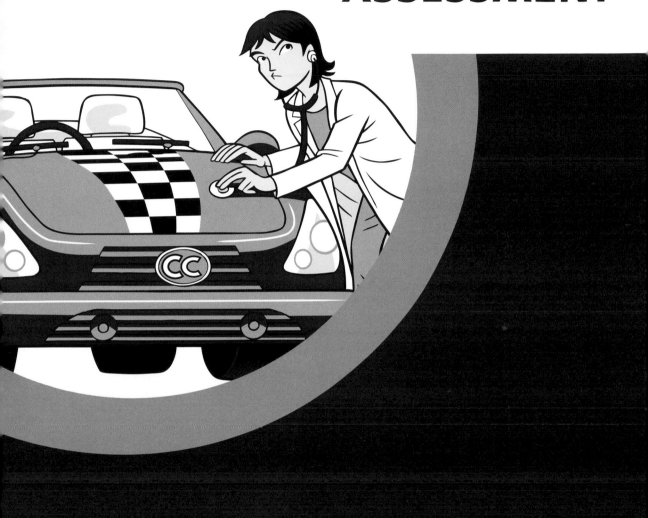

CLINICAL ASSESSMENT

Common presentations of cardiovascular disease

Objectives

You should be able to:

- List the questions that should be asked to fully characterize a patient's report of chest pain.
- Identify the most likely diagnosis given a description of chest pain.
- Recall the differential diagnosis of dyspnoea.
- Identify the common causes of hypertension and hypotension.
- Recognize the signs and symptoms of hyperlipidaemia.
- Understand the pathology of the various causes of syncope.
- Be aware of other signs and symptoms of cardiovascular disease, e.g. palpitations.
- Recognize the manifestations of peripheral vascular disease.
- Recognize the manifestations of diseases of the veins and lymphatics.
- Understand the management of cardiac arrest.

COMMON PRESENTING COMPLAINTS

Cardiovascular disease may present in a number of ways. Chest pain is the most obvious example, but shortness of breath or reduced exercise tolerance may be the first thing noticed by a patient. It should not be forgotten that some cardiovascular conditions may be asymptomatic, and these are diagnosed fortuitously when the patient is being examined for another complaint, or at a routine medical check-up.

In this chapter we will discuss the common presentations of cardiovascular disease, and the differential diagnoses that they infer.

The algorithms for presenting complaints are only a general guide to establishing a diagnosis. Many complaints may strongly indicate a particular diagnosis, but the patient might have a different problem – for example the patient may present with a burning central chest pain after eating; this may be indigestion, but it might be a mild myocardial infarction. Remember that medicine is not an exact science; you are always dealing in probability. The diagnosis will need to be confirmed by investigation (e.g. measuring levels of cardiac enzymes).

Chest pain

When a patient presents with chest pain (Figs 7.1 and 7.2), the following features must be elicited:

- Exact site, character and severity of pain.
- Onset and subsequent timing.
- Duration.
- Radiation (e.g. to the arms).
- Precipitating factors (e.g. exercise).
- Relieving factors (e.g. rest).
- Associated features.

Angina

Angina is characterized by a constricting, tightening, or choking pain on exertion that is relieved by rest or glyceryl trinitrate (GTN). The pain may radiate to the left arm and neck, and it may be exacerbated by emotion, large meals, or cold weather.

Acute coronary syndromes

Acute coronary syndromes include unstable angina or myocardial infarction. The myocardial infarction

Fig. 7.1 Causes of central and peripheral chest pain. These should be used as a guide only as ischaemia can present in many ways.

Causes of central and lateral chest pain	
Central pain	Lateral pain

Cardiac
   Angina
   Myocardial infarction
   Pericarditis
   Mitral valve prolapse
	Respiratory
	   Pneumonia
	   Pneumothorax
	   Neoplasia
	   Tuberculosis
	   Connective tissue disorders

Aortic
   Dissecting aortic aneurysm
   Aortitis
	Chest wall disorders
	(cause pleuritic pain)
	   Rib fracture
	   Intercostal muscle injury

Pulmonary/mediastinal
   Embolus
   Tracheitis
   Neoplasia
	Psychogenic
	   Anxiety

Oesophageal
   Oesophagitis (indigestion)
   Mallory–Weiss syndrome
	Other
	   Pulmonary embolus
	   Herpes zoster

Traumatic	
Psychogenic	

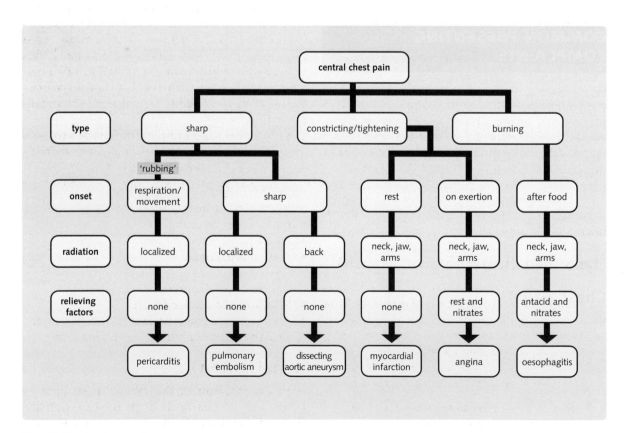

Fig. 7.2 Chest pain algorithm.

may be transmural (full thickness) or subendocardial (superficial). They are characterized by a spontaneous onset of continuous intense constricting or tightening pain at rest, which may be accompanied by sweating and vomiting. The patient may be very anxious and feel that he or she is about to die (sense of impending doom).

Acute ischaemia may also present very vaguely, known as silent ischaemia. This is most common in diabetics and the elderly, as denervation prevents the subjective feeling of pain.

Acute pericarditis

Acute pericarditis is characteristically described as a sharp pain, usually localized to the left of the sternum. It varies in intensity with movement and respiration.

Dissecting aortic aneurysm

A patient with a dissecting aortic aneurysm may present with severe, sharp, tearing pain radiating to the back. The pulses may be slow and asymmetrical.

Oesophageal spasm

Oesophageal pain often mimics angina – it may be precipitated by exercise, and it may be relieved with GTN. It may be described as a burning pain with a history related to food intake or oesophageal reflux.

Aortic stenosis and hypertrophic obstructive cardiomyopathy

These two conditions may also mimic angina. Symptomatic patients with these conditions warrant consideration for surgery.

Dyspnoea (shortness of breath)

Some key points need to be considered when attempting to identify the origin of dyspnoea. How short of breath is the patient? Is the dyspnoea brought on by exercise or is the patient short of breath at rest? What is the patient's exercise tolerance and functional reserve (ask about dressing, climbing stairs and walking)? Dyspnoea may be caused by:

- Heart failure if associated with orthopnoea, paroxysmal nocturnal dyspnoea (PND) or oedema.

- Mitral stenosis.
- Shock.
- Respiratory causes (e.g. asthma, pulmonary embolism, pneumothorax).

Orthopnoea

Orthopnoea is shortness of breath while lying flat. It indicates left heart failure. Ask the patient 'Can you lie flat to sleep?' 'Do you need to prop yourself up with pillows?' 'If so, how many?'

Paroxysmal nocturnal dyspnoea

Paroxysmal nocturnal dyspnoea (PND) is a sudden shortness of breath at night, causing the patient to awaken. It indicates left heart failure. Ask the patient 'Do you get attacks of breathlessness that wake you up at night?' 'How do you get your breath?'

Hypertension

The World Health Organization definition of hypertension is blood pressure higher than 140 mmHg systolic or 90 mmHg diastolic in the elderly (see p. 110). Blood pressure must be elevated on more than one examination for the patient to be diagnosed as hypertensive. If no organ damage is uncovered, then blood pressure measurements should be taken over a long period of time before a diagnosis of hypertension is reached. Mild hypertension is usually asymptomatic.

Secondary causes of hypertension are suggested by a specific history, e.g. sweating and tachycardia suggest phaeochromocytoma (see p. 113).

Malignant hypertension often presents with:

- Visual impairment.
- Nausea and vomiting.
- Fits.
- Transient paralysis.
- Severe headaches.
- Impairment of consciousness.
- Symptoms of cardiac failure.
- Angina (due to atherosclerosis or high oxygen demand from hypertrophied myocardium).

Hypotension

Hypotension results if the systolic blood pressure falls below 80 mmHg. It often presents with the classic features of shock (tachycardia and cold, clammy skin, etc.). Hypotension can be caused by:

- Anaphylactic, cardiogenic, or septicaemic shock.
- Volume depletion (hypovolaemic shock) – haemorrhage, burns, gastrointestinal losses (vomiting or diarrhoea), renal losses (diuretic therapy, nephropathy, diabetes mellitus).
- Drugs and drug overdose – opiates, barbiturates, amphetamines, antidepressants.

Commonly, postural hypotension occurs initially. This is a fall in blood pressure on standing >15 mmHg (blood pressure should normally rise because of venoconstriction in the legs). The causes of postural hypotension are:

- Volume depletion.
- Autonomic failure (caused by diabetes mellitus or amyloidosis).
- Drugs that interfere with autonomic function (e.g. ganglion blockers or tricyclic antidepressants).
- Interference with peripheral venoconstriction by drugs (e.g. nitrates, calcium antagonists, α-blockers).
- Prolonged bed rest.

Elevated serum cholesterol and triglycerides

Hyperlipidaemic patients may present with the following conditions or signs:

- Xanthoma (lipid deposits in a tendon).
- Xanthelasma or corneal arcus (lipid deposits in the cornea).
- Obesity.
- Hypertension.
- Pancreatitis.
- Diabetes mellitus.

Patients may also have a family history of lipid disorders or coronary heart disease. Secondary causes of hyperlipidaemia must be excluded. These include:

- Hypothyroidism.
- Diabetes mellitus.
- Obesity.
- Renal impairment.
- Nephrotic syndrome.
- Liver dysfunction.
- Dysglobulinaemia.
- Drugs (especially oral contraceptives, thiazides, corticosteroids).

Heart murmurs

If a patient with a heart murmur is cyanosed, a shunt may be present. Ask whether the patient can feel a thrill (a murmur you can palpate with your hand). Note whether the murmur is causing the patient any symptoms, e.g. dyspnoea, chest pain, fatigue.

Listen to the murmur in the auscultatory areas and decide where the murmur is in relation to the cardiac cycle. Listen for intensity, radiation, and any other associated sounds. Diastolic murmurs should be considered to be a serious sign. For more details and a differential diagnosis see Chapter 8.

Syncope (fainting)

Ask the patient whether they have ever fainted. The following points should be noted:

- Onset.
- Any loss of consciousness.
- Any warning (aura).
- Light-headedness or vertigo beforehand.
- Duration.
- Any memory loss.
- Any injuries sustained during the faint.
- Any incontinence or tongue biting.

  Syncope can be caused by:

- Vasovagal attack – a powerful centrally mediated reflex, initiated by pain, powerful emotional stimulus or sudden underperfusion of the brain (see Chapter 4).
- Stokes–Adams attack – a transient arrhythmia that causes a loss of cardiac output. Usually, there is no warning (but possible palpitation). It may cause pallor and an irregular or slow pulse.
- Aortic stenosis or intracardiac thrombus/ tumour – produces a similar picture.
- Postural hypotension – occurs when standing suddenly.
- Carotid sinus syndrome – occurs in patients aged over 50 years while turning their head. The carotid baroreceptors become extremely sensitive and are stimulated by gentle pressure. This can be checked for by massaging one of the carotids while feeling for extreme bradycardia.
- Vertebrobasilar insufficiency – also occurs while turning the head. The vertebral arteries running through the cervical spine often become pinched by bony spurs.

- Respiratory causes – cough syncope or anxiety with hyperventilation.
- Other causes – hypoglycaemia, raised intracranial pressure, or alcohol/drug ingestion. Epilepsy should also be considered.

Palpitation

Ask if the patient has ever had an episode of palpitation: 'Do you ever notice your heart beat?' 'Does it go really fast?' 'Can you tap it out on the table for me?' Palpitation is caused by:

- Arrhythmias. A regularly irregular pulse indicates intermittent heart block or ectopic beats; an irregularly irregular pulse indicates atrial fibrillation.
- Anxiety.

COMMON PRESENTING COMPLAINTS OF THE PERIPHERAL VASCULATURE

Oedema

Ask the patient 'Have you noticed any swelling in your feet or ankles?' Peripheral oedema is an indication of:

- Congestive cardiac failure – oedema indicates the characteristic fluid retention of heart failure.
- Venous thrombosis.
- Lymphoedema (caused by Milroy's syndrome, radiotherapy, malignancy or infection) if the oedema is non-pitting (i.e. when you press the skin, no indentation remains).
- Other diseases (e.g. liver disease, nephrotic syndrome, starvation etc.).

Intermittent claudication

Intermittent claudication is an indication of peripheral vascular disease impeding arterial flow in the legs. You should ask the patient 'Do you get cramp-like pain in your legs while walking or at rest?' 'How far can you walk?' 'How long do you have to rest to allow the pain to go away?' See p. 108 for more details.

A good method to use if you are stuck for a diagnosis is to employ a surgical sieve. This is a methodical approach to obtaining differential diagnoses by considering systems. Usually the first approach is to consider congenital and acquired causes. The acquired causes are further subdivided. A mnemonic for this is 'TIN CAN BED MID': T – trauma, I – infection, N – neoplasia, C – connective tissue disorders, A – autoimmune, N – nervous system, B – blood disorders, E – endocrine, D – drugs, M – metabolic disorders, I – idiopathic and iatrogenic, D – deficiency and degenerative.

Acute ischaemia

This may occur for several reasons:

- Acute decompensation of chronic ischaemia.
- Thrombosis in the vessel.
- Embolism.
- Trauma.

The most common presentation is that of an acutely cold, painful limb.

Ulceration and trophic changes

Many disorders of the cardiovascular system may present with either ulceration or trophic changes. See p. 161 for more details.

Veins and lymphatics

Varicose veins are often asymptomatic, but may present to clinics for cosmetic reasons. They may also cause an aching sensation, or bleed when knocked.

Deep venous thrombosis may be asymptomatic, present as calf swelling or as pulmonary embolism with chest pain.

Diseases of the lymphatics will usually present either at birth or shortly after if congenital, or with a subacute swelling of the limbs if acquired.

CARDIAC ARREST

Cardiac arrest occurs when there is an absence of cardiac output. Basic life support should be commenced immediately whilst the cardiac arrest team is called, and a cardiac monitor attached to the patient.

There are two main types of cardiac arrest, 'shockable' and 'non-shockable', referring to whether or not they respond to defibrillation. 'Shockable' rhythms include:

- Ventricular fibrillation – uncoordinated ventricular contraction.
- Ventricular tachycardia – broad complex tachycardia with no discernable output. 'Non-shockable' rhythms include:

- Pulseless electrical activity – the electrical activity of the heart is compatible with an output but there is no pulse; the obstruction is in some way mechanical.
- Asystole – an absence of cardiac electrical activity.

Once the type of cardiac arrest has been determined a strict algorithm is followed, as outlined in Fig 7.3.

Cardiac arrest into a 'shockable' rhythm is usually due to a cardiac cause. Defibrillation attempts to stop the abnormal electrical activity

Fig 7.3 Cardiac arrest algorithm (redrawn with permission from the Resuscitation Council of the United Kingdom – RCUK).

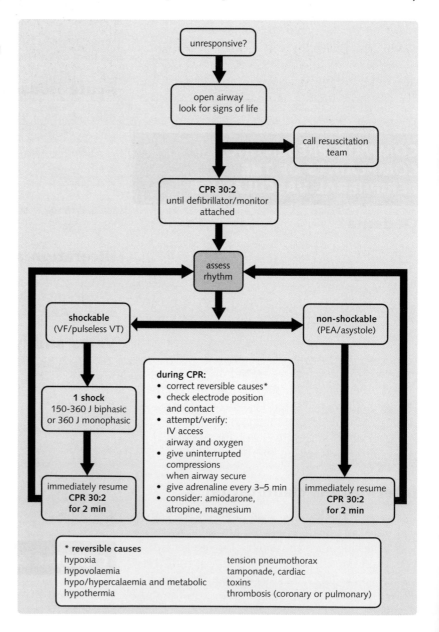

unresponsive?

open airway
look for signs of life

call resuscitation
team

CPR 30:2
until defibrillator/monitor
attached

assess
rhythm

shockable
(VF/pulseless VT)

non-shockable
(PEA/asystole)

1 shock
150-360 J biphasic
or 360 J monophasic

during CPR:
- correct reversible causes*
- check electrode position
  and contact
- attempt/verify:
  IV access
  airway and oxygen
- give uninterrupted
  compressions
  when airway secure
- give adrenaline every 3–5 min
- consider: amiodarone,
  atropine, magnesium

immediately resume
**CPR 30:2
for 2 min**

immediately resume
**CPR 30:2
for 2 min**

* reversible causes
hypoxia
hypovolaemia
hypo/hypercalaemia and metabolic
hypothermia

tension pneumothorax
tamponade, cardiac
toxins
thrombosis (coronary or pulmonary)

in the hope that the sinoatrial node will regain control.

Cardiac arrest into a 'non-shockable' rhythm is usually from a non-cardiac cause. These are divided into four 'H's and four 'T's:

- Hypovolaemia.
- Hypothermia.
- Hypotension.
- Hypo/hyperkalaemia and metabolic disturbances.
- Tension pneumothorax.
- Tamponade (pericardial).
- Thrombo-embolic.
- Toxic and therapeutic.

Whilst basic life support is being undertaken, consideration should be given to these reversible causes. Adrenaline and oxygen should be given to all patients. Atropine should be given to those patients in 'non-shockable' cardiac arrests where the ventricular rate is <60 bpm. Amiodarone should be given to those patients in 'shockable' cardiac arrests which are refractory to defibrillation, i.e. fail to respond to repeated cycles of shocks.

Cardiac arrests occur regularly in the hospital setting, although in a number of situations a 'Do Not Attempt Resuscitation' or 'DNR' order is put in place. These are written by senior members of staff when it is thought that death is expected, resuscitation under the circumstances would be futile, or the patient's quality of life subsequently would be very poor. These are obviously very difficult decisions to make, and a sound knowledge of ethical principles and medical law is essential.

History and examination

8

Objectives

You should be able to:

- Understand the principles of conducting a patient interview.
- Recall the specific questions to ask when conducting a focused cardiovascular system history.
- Understand the importance of observing the patient from the end of the bed.
- Recognize clinical signs in the hand and know their diagnostic inference.
- Describe how to palpate the peripheral pulses and be aware of abnormalities which may be found.
- Recognize clinical signs in the face and know their diagnostic inference.
- Understand the normal jugular venous pressure waveform and how this differs in disease.
- Conduct a thorough examination of the thorax.
- Understand the principles of auscultation of the heart, including heart sounds and murmurs.
- Recognize clinical signs in the abdomen and know their diagnostic inference.

TAKING A HISTORY

Important points to remember when taking a history include observation, introduction, and communication. These are discussed in more detail below.

Observation

Have a look around the bed for clues as to the patient's condition. (Are there inhalers on the bedside table? Are there walking aids in the room? Are there intravenous drips, oxygen bottles, or monitors?)

Make an initial assessment of the patient. (Is the patient in distress, finding it hard to breathe? How many pillows is the patient using?)

This assessment should continue and be updated throughout the interview.

Introduction

Always greet the patient and introduce yourself, explaining who you are and what you are about to do.

Ensure that the patient is comfortable at all times. Be prepared to halt the interview if circum-

stances warrant (e.g. the patient might want to go to the toilet, or lunch might arrive). Remember you can always come back later.

If there are relatives around, do not be afraid to ask them to leave to allow you to talk privately. Obviously, if the relative has only just got there or has only got a limited time with the patient, then you must come back at a more appropriate time.

If there are other people with the patient while you are taking a history (this can be daunting initially), you can use them to corroborate or give a collateral history of the information presented. Sensitive questions can be reserved until the examination when you will be alone with the patient.

Communication

Non-verbal communication

Sit down at a comfortable distance from the patient. Give the patient your full attention and make only brief notes.

Listen to what the patient is saying rather than just writing it down; you will then pick up on comments that can lead to further questions. This is harder than it sounds as frequently you are concentrating so hard on trying to think of the next question that you do not hear a vital clue. Keep the conversation flowing by nodding at appropriate moments, and using other non-verbal gestures.

Verbal communication

Initially ask open-ended questions ('What was the pain like?') rather than leading ones ('Was it a crushing pain?'). Closed questions ('What time did the pain start?') can be used later in the interview to clarify detail.

Let patients answer questions in their own words, without interruption. You should be aiming to hold a conversation rather than performing an interrogation. If you feel that the patient is rambling, gently try to steer the conversation back with a direct question ('If I could just clarify what the pain was like . . .?').

Try not to use medical terms (e.g. for orthopnoea, ask 'How many pillows do you need to get to sleep?').

If a patient says he has a certain condition, ask him to explain what he understands it to be and how it affects him. Beware of terms like 'gastric flu' or even 'angina'. What does the patient mean by this?

Use phrases like 'yes', 'a-ha', and 'I see' to help the conversation flow.

Overall, try to be friendly and confident and attempt to make the patient feel at ease. Do not be too worried if you cannot reach a diagnosis, but try to think of what the problem could be and commit yourself to a list of differential diagnoses and a management plan, no matter how simple.

Presenting complaint

The presenting complaint is a symptom reported by the patient and not a diagnosis. There may be more than one complaint; in which case, number the symptoms and take a history for each complaint.

History of the presenting complaint

Generally you need to find out the following information:

- Nature of the complaint.
- Site of the complaint.

- Extent of the deficit. How disabling is it?
- Onset. What time during the day? Which activities bring it on?
- Course. How does the symptom pattern vary? What is the frequency – is it intermittent or continuous?
- Duration. How long has it been there?
- Precipitating and relieving factors.
- Other relevant symptoms.
- Any previous treatment or investigations for this same complaint.

You should usually let the patient tell you the natural history of the complaint, but symptoms you should specifically ask about are:

- Chest pain.
- Shortness of breath, orthopnoea and paroxysmal nocturnal dyspnoea (PND).
- Oedema.
- Palpitation.
- Syncope (fainting) or dizziness.
- Intermittent claudication.
- Other symptoms – any coldness, redness or blueness of the extremities (symptoms of peripheral vascular disease); sweating; fever; appetite change, nausea, or vomiting (symptoms of heart failure or digitalis toxicity); tiredness (might be caused by heart failure or ischaemia, or may be a consequence of treatment such as β-blockers).

Risk factors

If the history is of ongoing ischaemic heart disease, it is also useful at this stage to make a list of risk factors which the patient does or does not have. See p. 78 to remind yourself of these.

Knowledge of these risk factors helps to formulate a management plan tailored specifically to that individual patient.

Review of systems

This is a systematic review of the whole body in an attempt to elicit any other symptoms. Points to note are outlined below.

Respiratory system

Note the presence of any cough, sputum or haemoptysis. This may indicate pulmonary oedema, and it is also a side effect of angiotensin-converting enzyme (ACE) inhibitors.

Gastrointestinal system

Epigastric pain might be caused by a myocardial infarction. Other abdominal pain might be caused by an aortic aneurysm (if it ruptures, there may be continuous abdominal pain) or ischaemia of the mesenteric vessels.

Genitourinary system

Causes of increased frequency of micturition and increased urine production include diabetes mellitus and diuretic therapy. Intermittent tachycardias may also cause increased urine production. Nocturia (needing to micturate at night) may be caused by heart failure.

Musculoskeletal system and skin

Joint pain can indicate a systemic disorder with cardiac effects (e.g. systemic lupus erythematosus).

Changes in the colour of the skin and the presence of rashes may also give vital clues to the underlying pathology.

Nervous system

A note should be made of:

- Any visual disturbances (e.g. amaurosis fugax – 'seeing curtains drawn across the eye').
- Temporary blindness (due to emboli reaching the retinal vessels and causing ischaemia of the retina – these emboli can arise from atheromatous plaques).
- Fits, faints, funny turns and funny sensations.

Systemic

This is very important and frequently omitted Knowledge of how the patient feels and the presence of systemic symptoms may give vital clues to the underlying diagnosis. Specific symptoms to ask about include:

- Eating – diet, appetite, weight loss.
- Sleeping – sleep disturbances, night sweats.
- Fever.
- Mood.

When taking a history it is important to individualize it to the patient in order to gain a holistic view. This is particularly important with risk factors for ischaemic heart disease, and how their angina limits their hobbies and activities.

Past medical history

Ask the patient if they have any other medical problems. Then say 'I'm going to run through a list of conditions to make sure we don't miss anything out – you might say "No" to most of these . . .'.

Important past medical conditions to note include:

- Diabetes mellitus.
- Hypertension.
- Myocardial infarction.
- Stroke (cerebrovascular accident – CVA).
- Angina.
- Arrhythmia.
- Peripheral vascular disease.
- Rheumatic fever.
- Intermittent claudication.
- Renal failure.

Follow this by asking about previous surgery. Specific procedures to note include:

- Coronary artery bypass graft (CABG).
- Angioplasty.
- Pacemakers and other implantable devices.
- Vascular surgery.

Drug history

A note should be made of all prescription and over-the-counter medications that are currently being used. The dose, preparation, frequency, route, compliance and adverse reactions to all these medications should be documented. It is important to remember that aspects of the presenting complaint may be due to current drug therapy. Be aware that some herbal and alternative medications have pharmacological effects or interactions (e.g. St John's wort and digoxin).

Any allergies should be noted, especially those due to drugs. To establish whether a true anaphylactic reaction takes place, ask the patient what happens when they come into contact with the substance.

Family history

Any relevant family history should be noted. Ask whether there is any incidence of the following diseases in close relatives:

- Diabetes mellitus.
- Myocardial infarction.
- CVA.
- Angina.
- Hypertension.
- Any hereditary disorder.

Find out the state of health of the patient's father, mother, siblings, and children. If they have died, ask what they died of and at what age, but remember to be sensitive.

A positive family history for myocardial infarction is <50 years for a male first-degree relative and <55 for a female first-degree relative.

Social history

This is a good opportunity to gain a holistic view of the patient, and place their disease in the context of their life. Enquire into the patient's marital status and whether they have children. Note the patient's present living conditions and any problems that these may cause (e.g. 'are there many steps that the patient cannot negotiate?'). Ask whether they manage with their activities of daily living (ADLs), e.g. washing, dressing, cooking, or whether they require assistance. Life-style factors, including diet and exercise, should be elicited:

- If the patient has ever smoked, find out how many per day, and for how many years. This can be used to calculate the number of pack years; one pack (20 cigarettes) per day for one year is one pack year.
- How much alcohol is consumed? How often? It is notoriously difficult to get an accurate history of alcohol consumption: often, you must ask questions like 'How long does a bottle of whisky last you?' Attempt to record this in units per week.
- Has the patient ever taken any illicit drugs?
- Ask if the patient has travelled abroad recently.

You might also need to ask about sexual practices.

A careful occupational history should not be neglected. Find out the patient's current and previous employment, with particular emphasis on levels of stress and industrial exposure to chemicals or physical agents. Be aware that patients may be worried about the consequences of their health on their job, and that there are medicolegal implications with certain careers (e.g. commercial driver, pilot).

OBSERVATION OF THE WHOLE PATIENT

General appearance

Note the general appearance of the patient. Is the patient:

- Well/ill/distressed?
- Alert/confused?
- Happy/sad?
- Thin/fat?

> Adopt a system for doing the examination. For example, always examine in the following order:
> - Inspection, then palpation, percussion, and auscultation of each area that you are examining.
> - Examine the hands, then the upper limbs, neck, face, chest, and abdomen; then, examine the lower limbs.

Colour

Look at the skin. Note any evidence of:

- Pallor/anaemia – pale skin.
- Cyanosis/shock – blueish tinge.
- Jaundice – yellowing of the skin.

These may imply:

- Hypovolaemia.
- Peripheral vascular disease.
- Pulmonary to systemic shunting.
- Lung disease.
- Haemoglobinopathy.

- Haemolytic conditions which may affect the heart.

Rash

Look at any rash. Note size, type [macula (flat) or papula (raised)], colour, surface, and reaction to pressure – does it blanch or not?

Gross abnormalities

Marfan syndrome

Marfan syndrome is usually an autosomal dominant inherited condition. Those with the syndrome show the following signs:

- Elongated and asymmetrical face.
- Dislocation of the lens of the eye (ectopia lentis).
- High-arched palate.
- Tall, with lower half of body larger than the upper half. The arm span is usually longer than the height.
- Long thin digits (arachnodactyly).

Degeneration of vessel media can lead to a dissecting aneurysm in the ascending aorta, which may rupture. An incompetent mitral and/or aortic valve may also result.

Down syndrome

Down syndrome is trisomy of chromosome 21. Those with the syndrome show the following signs:

- Large occiput, flat face with slanting eyes and epicanthic folds.
- Small ears.
- Simian crease (single plantar crease on the palm).
- Short, stubby fingers.
- Hypotonia.
- Sandal gap toes.

There is a variable level of mental retardation. Up to 50% of children with Down syndrome have a congenital heart defect, the most common being a ventricular septal defect, although atrioventricular septal defect is pathognomonic.

Turner's syndrome

In Turner's syndrome, the genotype is XO (phenotypically female). Those with the syndrome show infantilism (appear child-like even when an adult),
a webbed neck, short stature, cubitus valgus (increased carrying angle of elbow), and primary amenorrhoea (no menstrual bleeding).

Intelligence is normal. Other features can include coarctation of the aorta and other left-sided heart defects and lymphoedema of the legs.

THE UPPER LIMBS

Fig. 8.1 gives details about examination of the hands. Both hands should be inspected on the anterior and posterior aspects.

There are few signs to note in the arms and forearms. However, the radial and brachial pulses must be assessed (see below). Blood pressure should also be taken at this point.

Peripheral arterial pulses

Pulses should be checked as a matter of routine on all patients. Pulses on both sides of the body should be checked and compared.

Radial pulse

Palpate the radial pulse with the tips of the fingers and gently compress the radial artery against the head of the radius. This pulse is often used to assess heart rate and rhythm. The pulse character however is best assessed at the carotid. After locating the pulse, wait a while before counting the rate. The rate should be counted for about 30 s and then doubled to give a rate per minute. A normal pulse is between 60 and 100 beats per minute (bpm). Outside this range is bradycardia (<60 bpm) or tachycardia (>100 bpm). The rhythm may be regular or irregular; if it is irregular, note whether it is a repeating irregularity (regularly irregular) or is completely irregular (irregularly irregular):

- Regular. Normal rhythm – remember sinus arrhythmia is normal (an increased rate during inspiration).
- Regularly irregular. Commonly caused by ectopic systolic beats or second-degree heart block (see Chapters 5 and 9).
- Irregularly irregular. Usually caused by atrial fibrillation or multiple ectopic beats (see Chapter 5).

The volume of the pulse should be assessed. A low volume implies a decreased cardiac output. A

Palpation of the thorax		
Sign observed	**Test performed**	**Diagnostic inference**
Position of apex beat (Fig. 8.8)	Place hand across the chest and feel with the tips of your fingers for the lateral edge of the pulsating apex	—
—	If the apex beat is not palpable, turn the patient on to the left side and then palpate in the anterior axillary line	—
Prominent apex beat	—	Left ventricular hypertrophy
Displaced apex beat medially	—	Lung collapse; lung fibrosis
Displaced apex beat laterally apex beat more lateral	—	Left ventricular enlargement; pleural effusion; pneumothorax
Thrusting, displaced apex beat forceful and lateral, downward movement of apex	—	Volume overload: mitral/aortic incompetence
Sustained apex beat forceful and sustained impulse, which is not displaced	—	Pressure overload: aortic stenosis; hypertension; left ventricular hypertrophy
Failed detection of apex beat	—	Obesity; obstructed airways disease (overinflated); pleural effusion; pericardial effusion; dextrocardia (very rare)
Parasternal heave pulsation at left base of sternum	Palpate praecordium	Right ventricular hypertrophy
Other pulsations noted on observation (see above)	—	—
Tapping apex beat, palpable first heart sound	—	Mitral stenosis
Palpable second heart sound	—	Systemic or pulmonary hypertension
Thrills	Palpable murmurs, which feel like the purring of a cat	—
Systolic thrills in aortic area	—	Aortic stenosis
Systolic thrill at apex	—	Mitral regurgitation
Diastolic thrill	—	Mitral stenosis; aortic regurgitation (uncommon)

Fig. 8.7 Palpation of the thorax.

ness indicates cardiac enlargement or pericardial effusion. A reduced area of cardiac dullness may indicate hyperinflation of the lungs.

Auscultation

The stethoscope has two ends, the bell and the diaphragm (this is the larger, flatter end). The diaphragm is better for listening to higher pitched sounds; therefore, it is best for hearing:

- First and second heart sounds.
- Systolic murmurs.
- Aortic diastolic murmurs (aortic incompetence).
- Opening snap of valves.

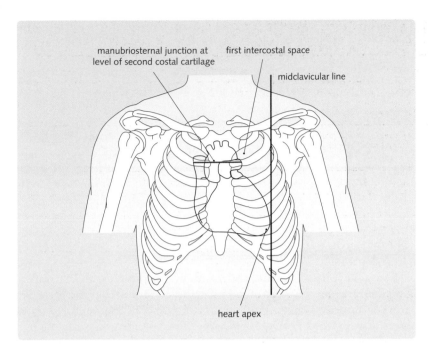

Fig. 8.8 Position of the apex beat. The apex beat is the position most inferior and furthest lateral that the cardiac impulse can be felt. As a guide to identifying intercostal spaces, the second rib lies lateral to the manubriosternal angle; the second intercostal space is below this rib. The lateral position can also be described relative to the anterior axillary line and the mid-axillary line. The normal apex beat lies in the fifth intercostal space, mid-clavicular line.

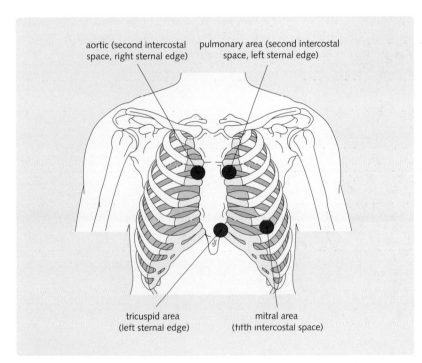

Fig. 8.9 Auscultatory areas. This shows where the valve sounds are best heard. These areas are not the surface markings of where the valves actually are (see Fig. 2.5).

The bell of the stethoscope is best for low-pitched sounds. The bell should not be placed too tightly to the skin, as it will then function as a diaphragm. It is used to hear:

- Third and fourth heart sounds.
- Mitral diastolic sounds (mitral stenosis).

There are certain areas where auscultation should be performed (Fig. 8.9); these are the areas where murmurs from heart valves are best heard:

- Mitral area (and axilla if murmur present).
- Tricuspid area.
- Aortic area (and neck if murmur present).

- Pulmonary area.
- The back.

Also use the diaphragm to auscultate the lungs to check for signs of pulmonary oedema (i.e. fine late inspiratory crackles).

Normal heart sounds

Many sounds can be heard with the stethoscope. Try to concentrate on hearing the heart sounds first, a repetitive 'lubb-dupp' (Fig 8.10). Auscultating while palpating the carotid pulse will help to distinguish the heart sounds.

The first heart sound (S_1) coincides with the onset of systole and, therefore, the pulse. It is caused by the closure of the mitral and tricuspid valves. S_1 is commonly labelled M_1T_1 to reflect its two sources. The second heart sound (S_2) coincides with the beginning of diastole and it is from the closure of the aortic and pulmonary valves. The components of S_2 are labelled A_2P_2. P_2 is only usually heard in the pulmonary area unless it is very loud.

Occasionally, the heart sounds may be split. This is when one component of the sound occurs before the other. For example, if the mitral valve (M_1) closes before the tricuspid (T_1) then S_1 is two distinct sounds, and it is said to be split.

S_1 is usually just one sound, and it is very rarely split. Any splitting of S_1 must not be mistaken for an ejection click or even S_4 (the fourth heart sound).

S_2 is normally split on inspiration (Fig. 8.11), especially in the young. Inspiration delays right heart emptying because it causes an increased venous return. This means the pulmonary valve is open longer and so closes later. Not all splitting of S_2 is normal however (Fig 8.12).

Abnormal heart sounds

The third and fourth heart sounds (S_3 and S_4, respectively) occur in diastole (Fig. 8.13), and they are caused by abnormal filling of the ventricle. S_3 is caused by passive filling in early diastole. S_4 is a consequence of atrial contraction, leading to an increased filling pressure.

S_3 is sometimes heard in healthy, young adults (younger than 35 years) and in pregnant women. Otherwise, the presence of S_3 indicates:

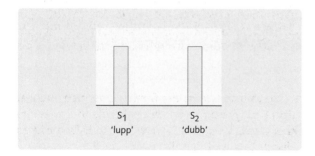

Fig. 8.10 Normal heart sound (S_1, first heart sound; S_2, second heart sound).

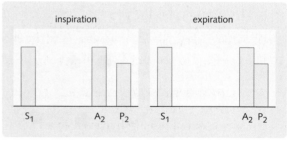

Fig. 8.11 Splitting of the second heart sound. S_2 may show physiological splitting into A_2 and P_2.

Fig. 8.12 Variations in the second heart sound. 'Fixed splitting' occurs when the second heart sound is split irrespective of respiratory movements; 'physiological splitting' refers to the normal splitting of S_2 with respiration and 'reverse splitting' occurs when the normal changes with respiration are reversed.

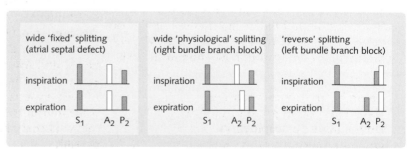

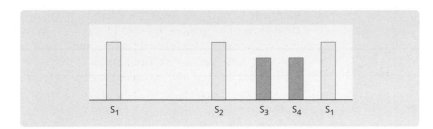

Fig. 8.13 The third and fourth heart sounds. The third heart sound creates a triple rhythm; the fourth heart sound is usually heard just before S_1 (da-lubb-dupp).

- Heart failure.
- Mitral regurgitation.
- Constrictive pericarditis (the high-pitched 'pericardial knock').

The presence of S_4 indicates a ventricle with decreased compliance (e.g. due to aortic stenosis or hypertension).

Clicks can be heard when abnormal aortic (e.g. in aortic stenosis) or pulmonary valves open. They are called ejection systolic clicks, and they occur in early systole – it sounds as if the first heart sound is split. Similar sounds occur with abnormal mitral or tricuspid valves where the sound is mid-diastolic and called an opening snap.

Alterations in sound intensity can indicate disease, for example:

- S_1 is loud in mitral stenosis.
- S_1 is soft in mitral regurgitation and first-degree heart block.
- S_1 is variable in second-degree heart block and atrial fibrillation.
- A_2 is loud in systemic hypertension.
- A_2 is soft in aortic stenosis.
- P_2 is loud in pulmonary hypertension.
- P_2 is soft in pulmonary stenosis.

Murmurs

Murmurs are caused by turbulent blood flow at a valve or an abnormal communication within the heart. The presence of a murmur does not always indicate disease, and the loudness does not always correlate with severity. Many individuals have innocent murmurs, called flow murmurs. These typically:

- Are soft, early systolic murmurs.
- Have a musical or grunting component.
- Do not have a palpable thrill.
- Occur in the young or the elderly.

- Occur in conditions with increased blood flow (e.g. anaemia, thyrotoxicosis, hypertension, pregnancy).

Murmurs are classified according to when they are heard (i.e. systolic, diastolic or continuous) (Fig. 8.14).

When auscultating cardiac murmurs, one of the most important distinctions to make is whether the murmur is systolic or diastolic – this can easily be determined by timing the murmur with the carotid pulse. Murmurs should be described by their site, timing, character, loudness and radiation. When a patient is found to have a murmur, they should have a minimum investigation including an ECG and echocardiogram.

Systolic murmurs are further classified into ejection (mid) systolic (intensity builds to a peak and then subsides before S_2) or pansystolic (same intensity throughout systole right up to S_2).

Diastolic murmurs are classified into early (shortly after or merging with S_2) or late (shortly before or merging with S_1).

Murmurs are sometimes very difficult to hear when you are first starting out; it is best to try to differentiate whether the murmur is systolic or diastolic. It is most likely to be systolic, and timing the murmur with a thumb on the carotid artery may be helpful. After this, try to differentiate between ejection systolic and pansystolic.

Even experts have difficulty in distinguishing some murmurs. Take every opportunity to hear as many normal hearts and obvious murmurs as possible.

Classification of cardiac murmurs			
Timing	Cause	Best heard	Radiates
Systolic murmurs: Ejection systolic S_1 S_2 S_1	Aortic stenosis Pulmonary stenosis Atrial septal defect Outflow tract obstruction	Aortic area Left sternal edge Left sternal edge —	Neck Loudest on inspiration — —
Pansystolic S_1 S_2 S_1 Late systolic	Mitral regurgitation (blowing) Tricuspid regurgitation (low-pitched) Ventricular septal defect (loud and rough) Mitral valve prolapse Coarctation of aorta Hypertrophic obstructive cardiomyopathy	Apex Left sternal edge Left sternal edge Apex Left sternal edge —	Axilla — — — — —
Diastolic murmurs: Mid-diastolic S_1 S_2 S_1	Mitral stenosis (low rumbling) Tricuspid stenosis Austin–Flint	Apex Left sternal edge Apex	Louder with exercise — —
Early diastolic S_1 S_2 S_1	Aortic regurgitation (blowing, high-pitched) Pulmonary regurgitation Graham–Steel in pulmonary hypertension	Left sternal edge Right sternal edge —	— — —
Continuous murmurs: S_1 S_2 S_1 Combined systolic and diastolic murmurs	Patent ductus arteriosus (machinery) Aortic stenosis and regurgitation	Left sternal edge Left sternal edge	— Neck
Venous hum	High venous flow especially in young children High mammary blood flow in a pregnant woman	Neck —	Reduced while lying flat —
Pericardial friction rub	Inflamed pericardium; scratching or crunching noise	—	Loudest in systole

Fig. 8.14 Types of cardiac murmur.

ABDOMEN

Inspection

Fig. 8.15 describes inspection of the abdomen for scars and skin lesions, and Fig. 8.16 shows how to tell the direction of venous flow. Again, it is important to observe the whole of the abdomen, which may involve the patient moving their arms.

Palpation

The abdomen should initially be palpated superficially to detect any tenderness, and then deeply to detect any masses, pulsations or organomegaly. Carefully palpate around all four quadrants of the abdomen. Fig. 8.17 describes some abnormalities which may be detected on palpation.

Percussion

Percussion can be used to outline the liver. If the liver edge cannot be felt then percuss over the right side. If there is dullness throughout, the liver may be so enlarged that it occupies the whole area. The alternative may be an abdomen distended with fluid, called ascites. If ascites is present there will be a fluid thrill and the dullness will shift when the patient is rolled onto their side.

Inspection of the abdomen for scars and skin lesions		
Sign observed	Test performed	Diagnostic inference
Dilated veins visible	Check direction of blood flow by pressing vein and watching direction of refilling (Fig. 8.16)	If flow of blood is superior: inferior vena caval obstruction If blood flow is inferior: superior vena caval obstruction If blood flow is radiating from umbilicus: portal vein obstruction
Pulsations in the epigastric region		Abdominal aortic aneurysm; visible peristalsis

Fig. 8.15 Inspection of the abdomen for scars and skin lesions.

push down on vein   push fingers apart   lift one finger and see if vein fills; if it does then blood is flowing from the lifted finger

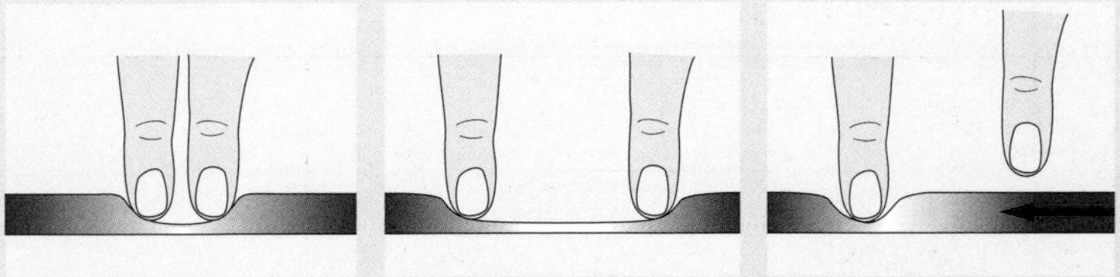

Fig. 8.16 Assessing direction of venous flow.

Fig. 8.17 Palpation of the abdomen.

Palpation of the abdomen		
Sign observed	Test performed	Diagnostic inference
Enlarged liver edge	Palpate right upper quadrant; feel liver edge by using the edge of your right hand and placing it deep; start low down and work your way up; ask the patient to breathe deeply	Right heart failure; infection; excess alcohol
Pulsatile liver edge	—	Tricuspid valve incompetence
Midline pulsatile mass	Palpate the epigastrium	Abdominal aortic aneurysm

A 47-year-old male comes in with a distended, fluid-filled abdomen. There are many causes to consider here, and these are divided into transudates (<30 g/dL protein) and exudates (>30 g/dL protein). Transudates are usually present as a result of pressure changes, e.g. an increased hydrostatic pressure in heart failure, or a decreased colloid osmotic pressure in nephrotic syndrome and protein-losing states. Exudates are usually inflammatory or neoplastic. The protein content of the fluid can be determined by taking a small sample, in this case an ascitic tap.

Auscultation

Auscultate over the abdomen listening for bowel sounds. If you suspect an abdominal aortic aneurysm, then auscultate over it to detect any bruits.

THE LOWER LIMBS

Many clues can be gained about pathology of the cardiovascular system from the condition of the lower limbs.

Arterial examination of the lower limbs

Area	Sign observed	Test performed	Diagnostic inference
Skin	Skin thinning, loss of hair, cold limbs	Observation	Arterial insufficiency
Heel of foot and between toes	Ulceration (well demarcated)	Assess if painful (arterial ulcers are, neuropathic ulcers are not)	Chronic arterial insufficiency
Lower limb	Venous guttering, white → blue → red discolouration	Buerger's test - raise limbs to ~ 30°, hold for 2 minutes and observe, lower the limbs over the edge of the bed	Critical ischaemia
Sites of arterial pulses (see text)	Absent or diminished pulses	Palpation and auscultation for bruits	Arterial insufficiency

Fig 8.18 Arterial examination of the lower limbs.

Venous examination of the lower limbs			
Area	**Sign observed**	**Test performed**	**Diagnostic inference**
Lower limbs	Varicose veins (distended, tortuous veins; usually affects the saphenous veins)	Assess if they are hard (thrombosed) or tender (phlebitis) by palpation	Thrombophlebitis may indicate a deep vein occlusion; prolonged standing
Ankle	Oedema	Press one finger in one place for one minute; see if the impression disappears quickly (normal) or not (pitting oedema)	Fluid retention Congestive cardiac failure Lymphoedema Deep vein occlusion Liver disease Nephrotic syndrome
Gaiter area ulceration	Ulcers (breakdown of the skin that becomes very difficult to heal). Venous ulcers are found around the medial malleolus (Gaiter area) Xanthomas (itchy, yellow, eruptive nodules with red edge on extensor surfaces e.g. buttocks) Tendon xanthomas on extensor tendons Cayenne pepper discolouration, atrophie blanche, hyperpigmentation, champagne bottling of legs	—	Deep vein occlusion Sickle cell anaemia Diabetes mellitus Vasculitides (polyarteritis nodosum) Squamous cell carcinoma skin lesion Hypertriglyceridaemia Lipoprotein lipase deficiency Familial hypercholesterolaemia Deep venous insufficiency
Lower limbs	Variosities in the distribution of the long saphenous (medial side) and/or short saphenous (lateral side) veins	Trendelenburg test; lie patient down and raise leg; place two fingers 5 cm below femoral pulse (sapheno-femoral junction); get patient to stand with fingers still in place; If veins do not fill, pressure over the area is compensating for an incompetent valve	Incompetent sapheno-femoral junction valve (may be amenable to surgery)

Fig. 8.19 Venous examination of the lower limbs.

Peripheral pulses

An examination of the peripheral pulses of the limbs should first start with inspection. The signs of peripheral vascular disease are shown in Fig. 8.18. You should then assess temperature, capillary refill time and the peripheral pulses by palpation. Auscultation should be performed over the vessels to assess for the presence of a bruit.

Femoral pulse

The femoral pulse is located just below the mid-inguinal point (half way between the anterior superior iliac spine and the pubic symphysis). It is a strong pulse and should be easy to palpate.

Popliteal pulse

The popliteal arteries can be found in the popliteal fossae behind the knee and are very hard to palpate.

The thumbs of both hands should be rested on either side of the patella and the fingertips should be placed deep into the popliteal fossa. The popliteals are best palpated with the knees flexed at about 120°.

Posterior tibial pulse

The posterior tibial pulse is palpated about 1 cm behind the medial malleolus of the tibia with the patient's foot relaxed.

Dorsalis pedis pulse

The dorsalis pedis pulse is palpated against the tarsal bones on the dorsum of the foot, just lateral to the tendon of extensor hallucis longus.

Examination of the venous system

Examination of the veins of the leg should be conducted with the patient standing, as varicosities, ulcers and trophic changes are usually more obvious. The signs of venous disease are described in Fig 8.19.

Ulceration often occurs on the lower limbs, and distinguishing between the different causes clinically is often very difficult. Arterial ulcers are usually deep, punched out lesions on the lateral aspect of the foot, between the toes and on pressure points. Venous ulcers are most often sloughy, and on the medial aspect of the calf in the gaiter area. The key to detecting neuropathic ulceration is to test the sensation in the feet. Diabetic ulcers tend to be a mixture of neuropathic and micro-angiopathic ulcers.

Investigations and imaging

Objectives

You should be able to:

- Explain the concept of the cardiac dipole, unipolar and dipolar leads.
- Conduct an ECG examination on a patient.
- Sketch a 'typical' ECG trace, showing the normal wave and normal parameters.
- Be familiar with common abnormalities in heart rate, rhythm and axis.
- Understand the role of echocardiography and the indications for its use.
- Recall the changes in cardiac enzymes associated with myocardial infarction.
- Understand the role of cardiac catheterization and Doppler ultrasonography.
- Understand the rationale for routine blood tests in patients with cardiovascular disease.
- Identify common lesions on plain chest radiographs.
- Identify CT, MRI, ultrasound and VQ scans.

INVESTIGATION OF CARDIOVASCULAR FUNCTION

Electrocardiography

The electrocardiogram (ECG) is a recording of the electrical activity of the heart, obtained by measuring the changes in electrical potential difference across the body. It is usually the first investigation used to diagnose arrhythmias and the underlying cause of chest pain.

The electrical signal that activates contraction of the myocytes creates a wave of depolarization. As the wave of depolarization spreads through the ventricle there will be, at any one moment, areas of the ventricle that have been excited and areas that have not yet been excited. In effect, there is a difference in potential between them: one area is negative in charge, the other is positive. These areas can be thought of as two electrical poles. This is the cardiac dipole (Fig. 9.1). This dipole depends on both the size of the charge (which depends on the amount of muscle excited) and the direction the wave of depolarization is travelling in. Recording electrodes are placed in certain positions on the body so that the cardiac dipole and other changes in potential can be measured in different directions.

Conventionally, the ECG is recorded using 12 leads (Fig. 9.2). Note that the term 'lead' is used to denote the direction in which the potential is measured and not a physical electrode – only 9 electrodes are used to produce the 12 leads. The additional 3 lead traces are produced using the 'standard leads', which show the potential difference between specific pairs of unipolar leads. These leads allow us to view the electrical activity in both the frontal (I, II, III, aVR, aVL, and aVF) and transverse (V$_1$ to V$_6$) planes, and in any direction in these planes.

Unipolar leads

Unipolar leads measure any positive potential difference directed towards their solitary electrode. These include:

- aVL, aVR, and aVF electrodes on both arms and the left leg. They view the heart in the frontal plane.
- Six chest electrodes labelled V$_1$ to V$_6$ – these measure any potential changes in the transverse plane, and they are arranged around the left side of the chest.

Standard leads

The potential difference shown by these leads is conventionally measured from:

- Lead I – right arm (aVR) to left arm (aVL); left arm positive.
- Lead II – right arm (aVR) to left leg (aVF); left leg positive.

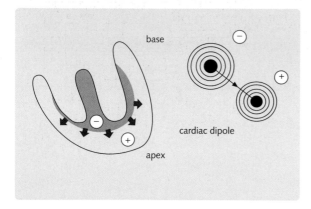

Fig. 9.1 The cardiac dipole. As the wave of depolarization travels from the atrioventricular (AV) node to the apex and base of the heart, it can be considered to move from an area of negative charge to an area of positive charge. The direction of the dipole at any time indicates how the wave of depolarization travels through the ventricle. (The area that has been excited is termed as 'negative' and the area to be excited as 'positive'. This reflects the changes in the charge in the extracellular space.)

- Lead III – left arm (aVL) to left leg (aVF); left leg positive.

These bipolar limb leads view the heart in the frontal plane. These three electrodes make up Eint-hoven's triangle around the heart (see below).

Remember that as the dipole has both charge (amplitude) and direction, the shape of the ECG varies depending upon the position of the recording electrode. The directions measured in the frontal plane and the associated changes in the ECG trace are shown in Fig. 9.3.

Normal electrocardiogram

The classical ECG trace is shown in Fig. 9.4. The elements of an ECG are:

- P wave – due to atrial depolarization.
- PR interval – from the onset of the P wave to the onset of the QRS complex (approximately 120–200 ms). This represents the time taken for atrial depolarization and the impulse to conduct through the AV node, His bundle and into the Purkinje fibres.
- QRS complex – due to ventricular depolarization (<120 ms).

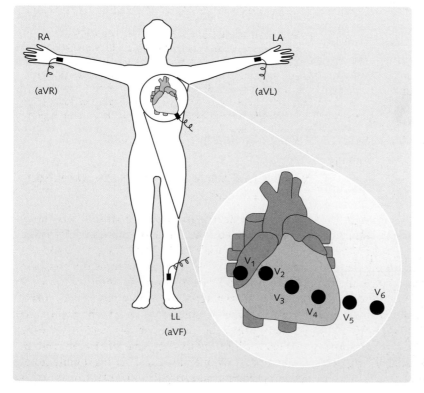

Fig. 9.2 Placement of electrocardiographic electrodes. The electrodes on the right arm (RA), left arm (LA), and left leg (LL) give the electrocardiogram trace for the frontal leads (i.e. I, II, III, aVL, aVR, and aVF). V_1 is placed in the fourth intercostal space on the left sternal edge, and V_2 on the right sternal edge. V_4 is placed in the fifth intercostal space in the mid-clavicular line, V_5 in the anterior axillary line, and V_6 in the mid-axillary line. V_3 is placed between V_2 and V_4.

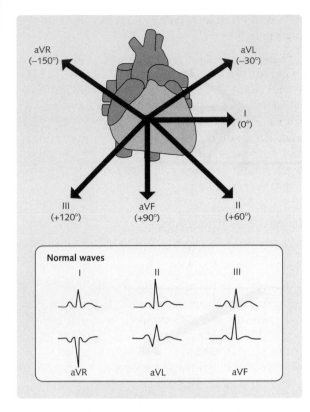

Fig. 9.3 Lead directions in the anterior plane. (Redrawn with permission from Epstein O et al. Clinical examination, 2nd edn. New York: Mosby International, 1997.)

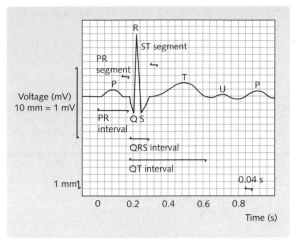

Fig. 9.4 Normal electrocardiogram.

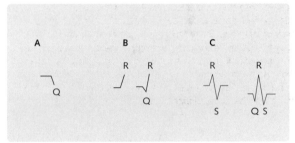

Fig. 9.5 Definitions of the ECG waves. If the wave following the P wave is negative, it is a Q wave (A). If a positive deflection follows the P wave, it is called an R wave, whether it is preceded by a Q wave or not (B). Any following negative deflection is known as an S wave, whether there has been a preceding Q wave or not (C). Abnormally large Q waves have an additional pathological significance (see Fig. 9.12).

- QT interval – the time taken from depolarization of the ventricles to the end of repolarization (approximately 400 ms).
- T wave – due to ventricular repolarization.

Note that the different components of the QRS complex are formally defined (Fig. 9.5).

ECG parameters simply need to be committed to memory! They are as follows:
- PR interval – approximately 120–200 ms.
- QRS duration – approximately 80 ms (but not usually more than 100 ms).
- QT duration – approximately 400 ms.

Why the T wave is in the same direction as the R wave

The wave of depolarization travels from the AV node down to the apex and base of the heart. This is the cause of the R wave in the ECG. If repolarization of the heart then took place in the same direction the T wave would be in the opposite direction to the R wave. However, repolarization actually takes place from the base of the heart towards the top of the septum. Thus, the wave of repolarization is in the opposite direction to the wave of depolarization, and so the T wave is upright. This is a double negative: repolarization is negative depolarization and it occurs in a negative direction, so it appears as if it is positive.

Cardiac axis

The average direction of the wave of depolarization is the electrical axis of the heart, referred to as the cardiac axis (Fig. 9.6). It must be established whether this is normal or not. There are three ways this can be established.

When the depolarization wave in the ventricles is moving towards a lead, then the R wave will be larger than the S wave in that lead. When the ventricular depolarization wave is moving away from a lead, then the S wave will be larger than the R wave in that lead. If the S wave and R wave are equal then the depolarization is moving (on average) at right angles to that lead.

Therefore, to assess the axis, find the lead in the frontal plane with the greatest R wave. The cardiac axis is generally in this direction. Also check that the lead which measures at right angles to this has an R and S wave that are approximately equal.

An alternative method is to count the maximum height of the QRS complex in leads I and aVF and plot this point on a graph with the axes being I (as the x-axis) and aVF (as the y-axis). Draw a line from the origin to this point. This reflects the axis of the heart (Fig. 9.6). This is an analysis of vectors with amplitude and direction (as in the parallelogram of forces). A similar approach is used when drawing Einthoven's triangle (Fig. 9.6).

The cardiac axis should be between +90° and −30° as shown in Fig. 9.3. Any deviation from this is abnormal and is termed right or left axis deviation.

Right axis deviation (axis more than +90°) is caused by:

- Right ventricular hypertrophy.
- Congenital heart disorders.

Left axis deviation (axis less than −30°) is caused by left ventricular hypertrophy.

Anterior chest leads (V₁–V₆)

The anterior chest leads look at the chest in the horizontal (or transverse) plane. The wave of depolarization in the ventricles starts in the septum and then spreads into the left and right ventricles (Fig. 9.7). Because the left ventricle is usually larger than the right, the average depolarization heads towards

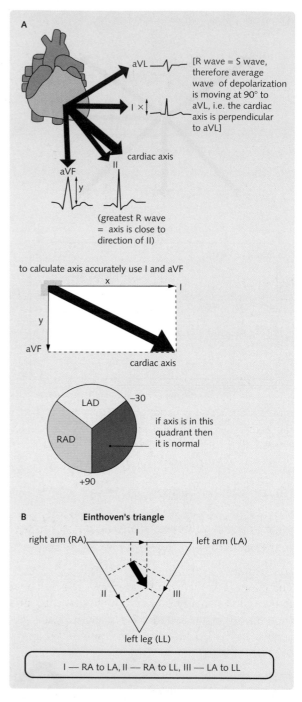

Fig. 9.6 (A) Normal axis and the different methods to measure it. (B) Einthoven's triangle. (LAD, left axis deviation; RAD, right axis deviation).

the left ventricle. This means that V_1 and V_2 will have a predominant S wave (i.e. negative deflection) and a small R wave, while V_5 and V_6 will have a predominant R wave (i.e. positive deflection) with a small S

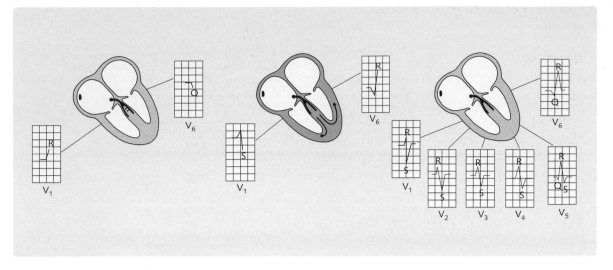

Fig. 9.7 The different anterior chest leads show different QRS traces due to the changing directions of the electrical activity. Lead V_4 is usually over the interventricular septum, and therefore usually shows equal R and S waves. Note the changing relative heights of Q, R, and S waves between leads. The changing height of the R wave from V_1 to V_6 is known as 'R wave progression'.

wave. The interventricular septum lies where there are equal positive and negative deflections (i.e. R and S waves), and is usually at V3 or V4. This steady increase in the size of the R wave is sometimes termed R wave progression. If this is normal then there is said to be 'good' R wave progression.

Rhythm disturbance

Rhythm disturbance is best assessed by looking at a long trace of lead II, which is often the closest lead to the cardiac axis.

Assessment of rate
The paper speed is usually 25 mm/s, which means that in 1 s the paper has moved by five large squares (i.e. 0.2 s per large square). Every small square represents 0.04 s. The rate can be measured in a variety of ways:

- Divide 300 by the number of large squares between QRS complexes. That will give you a rate in beats per minute.
- Find the time interval between R waves by multiplying the number of little squares by 0.04. Divide 60 s by this time interval to give a rate.
- If the interval between R waves is 1 large square the rate is 300 beats/min; 2 large squares, 150 beats/min; 3 large squares, 100

beats/min; 4 large squares, 75 beats/min; 5 large squares, 60 beats/min; 6 large squares, 50 beats/min (i.e. divide 300 by the number of large squares between beats).

Assessment of rhythm
Note whether the rhythm is regular, and whether every QRS complex is preceded by a P wave.

Note whether the PR interval is the same throughout. If the rhythm is irregular, is it irregularly irregular (e.g. atrial fibrillation) or regularly irregular (e.g. 2nd degree heart block)?

Arrhythmias

Heart block
Fig. 9.8 details the electrocardiographic appearance of the heart blocks.

Bundle branch block
Delay in the conduction system of the interventricular septum leads to widening of the QRS complexes (>0.12 s) (Fig. 9.9). Looking at leads V_1 and V_6 in right bundle branch block there is:

- A second R wave (R') in V_1 and a deeper, wider S wave in V_6.
- The last part of the QRS in lead V_1 is negative. This is because of the delayed right ventricular depolarization.

Fig. 9.8 Classification of heart blocks. Note that only the large squares of the ECG are shown for clarity.

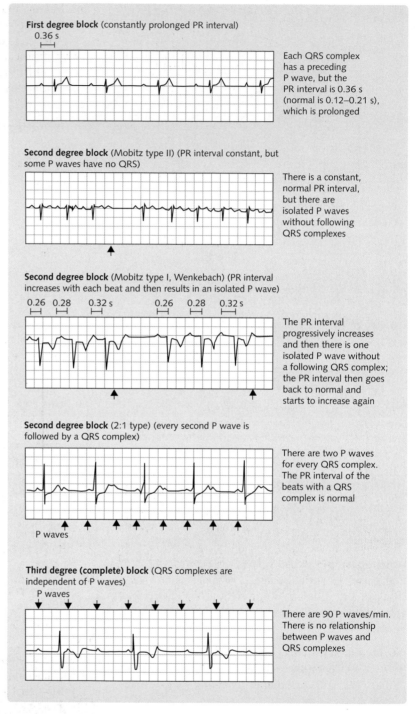

First degree block (constantly prolonged PR interval)

0.36 s

Each QRS complex has a preceding P wave, but the PR interval is 0.36 s (normal is 0.12–0.21 s), which is prolonged

Second degree block (Mobitz type II) (PR interval constant, but some P waves have no QRS)

There is a constant, normal PR interval, but there are isolated P waves without following QRS complexes

Second degree block (Mobitz type I, Wenkebach) (PR interval increases with each beat and then results in an isolated P wave)

0.26 0.28 0.32 s   0.26 0.28 0.32 s

The PR interval progressively increases and then there is one isolated P wave without a following QRS complex; the PR interval then goes back to normal and starts to increase again

Second degree block (2:1 type) (every second P wave is followed by a QRS complex)

There are two P waves for every QRS complex. The PR interval of the beats with a QRS complex is normal

P waves

Third degree (complete) block (QRS complexes are independent of P waves)

P waves

There are 90 P waves/min. There is no relationship between P waves and QRS complexes

This change can also be seen in lead I, where the last part of the QRS is negative due to the delayed right ventricular depolarization.

In left bundle branch block:

- There is a Q wave with an S wave in V_1.
- There is a notched R wave in V_6.

- The last part of the QRS in lead V_1 is positive. This reflects the delayed depolarization of the left ventricle.

Again, the delayed depolarization is also reflected in lead I, where the last section of the QRS shows a positive split peak.

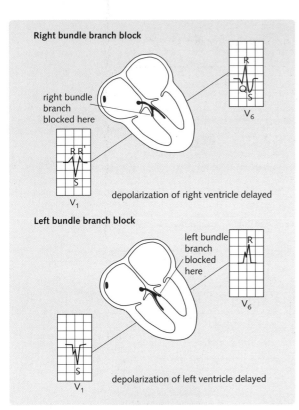

Right bundle branch block

right bundle branch blocked here

V_6

depolarization of right ventricle delayed

V_1

Left bundle branch block

left bundle branch blocked here

V_6

depolarization of left ventricle delayed

V_1

Fig. 9.9 Left and right bundle branch blocks. Disruption of the conduction system delays activation of ventricular muscle producing a characteristic split peak in the ECG.

To determine the type of bundle branch block, look at leads V_1 and V_6 and think of WiLLiaM MaRRoW. In LBBB, there is a W pattern in lead V_1, and an M pattern in V_6 (WiLLiaM). In RBBB, there is an M pattern in lead V_1, and a W pattern in V_6 (MaRRoW).

Atrial and ventricular rhythm disturbances

Electrocardiographic appearances of atrial and ventricular rhythm disturbances are shown in Figs 9.10 and 9.11.

Myocardial infarction

Electrocardiographic changes after myocardial infarction (Fig. 9.12) include:

- Within hours – ST elevation, and T wave lengthens and gets taller.

- Within 24 hours – T wave inversion, and ST elevation resolves.
- Within hours or days – abnormal large Q waves (indicating full thickness infarction) start to form and usually persist, T wave inversion may persist, ST segment returns to normal.

The leads in which these changes occur reflect the area of the heart affected:

- II, III, and aVF for an inferior infarct.
- V_1–V_4 for an anteroseptal infarct.
- V_4–V_6, I, and aVL for an anterolateral infarct.

In subendocardial infarction:

- There is T wave inversion.
- No Q waves form.

In true posterior infarct there is:

- A prominent R wave in V_2.
- ST depression.
- An upright T wave.

A 59-year-old gentleman with a history of ischaemic heart disease presents to the emergency department with chest pain. He is treated initially with oxygen, nitrates, morphine and aspirin whilst a 12-lead ECG is taken. It is important to interpret the ECG at an early stage, commenting on the following things:

- Name, age, and sex of the patient.
- Date and time the electrocardiogram was taken.
- Rate.
- Rhythm.
- Axis.

Next, note any abnormalities and in which lead they occur:

- P waves: width and height.
- PR interval.
- QRS complex: width and height.
- QT interval.
- ST segment.
- T waves: negative/positive and height.
- U waves.

After interpreting the ECG, provide an opinion and formulate a management plan.

Fig. 9.10 Atrial rhythm disturbances. These are also termed supraventricular arrhythmias.

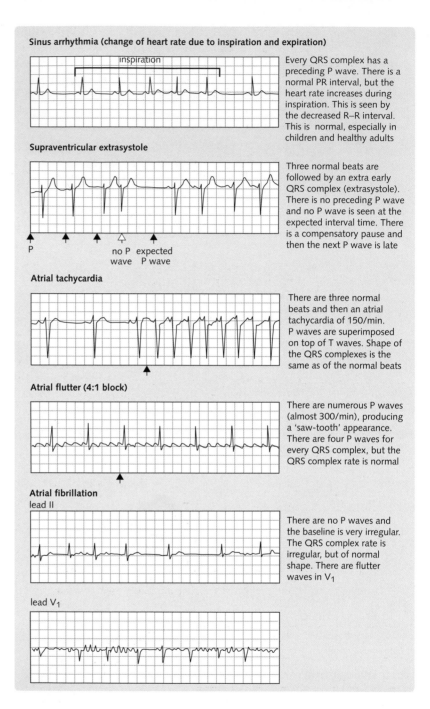

Sinus arrhythmia (change of heart rate due to inspiration and expiration)

Every QRS complex has a preceding P wave. There is a normal PR interval, but the heart rate increases during inspiration. This is seen by the decreased R–R interval. This is normal, especially in children and healthy adults

Supraventricular extrasystole

Three normal beats are followed by an extra early QRS complex (extrasystole). There is no preceding P wave and no P wave is seen at the expected interval time. There is a compensatory pause and then the next P wave is late

P   no P expected wave P wave

Atrial tachycardia

There are three normal beats and then an atrial tachycardia of 150/min. P waves are superimposed on top of T waves. Shape of the QRS complexes is the same as of the normal beats

Atrial flutter (4:1 block)

There are numerous P waves (almost 300/min), producing a 'saw-tooth' appearance. There are four P waves for every QRS complex, but the QRS complex rate is normal

Atrial fibrillation
lead II

There are no P waves and the baseline is very irregular. The QRS complex rate is irregular, but of normal shape. There are flutter waves in V_1

lead V_1

Electrocardiographic exercise test

An exercise or stress electrocardiogram is used to assess cardiac function in exercise. It is often used to diagnose angina and helps to provide prognostic information and inform future management. ST depression on an exercise electrocardiogram suggests myocardial ischaemia. This may also be found in ventricular hypertrophy and abnormal ventricular conduction.

Fig. 9.11 Ventricular rhythm disturbances.

Ventricular extrasystole (extraventricular beat)

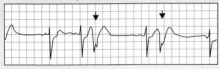

There are five sinus beats and then a ventricular extrasystole occurs, which is a wide QRS complex with an abnormal T wave.

Ventricular extrasystole with R on T phenomenon

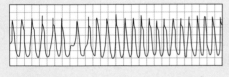

In this phenomenon the extrasystole beats occur on the T wave of the previous beat. It is said to be an 'R on T' phenomenon (i.e. an R wave on top of a T wave).

Ventricular tachycardia

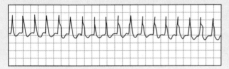

The rate of QRS complexes is almost 300/min. The QRS complexes are wide and abnormal in shape. There are no preceding P waves. This can often lead to ventricular fibrillation.

Paroxysmal tachycardia (sometimes called junctional tachycardia)

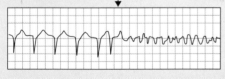

Rate is increased at 200/min, but there are preceding P waves and normal-shaped QRS complexes, which are slightly wider than normal due to a rate-related bundle branch block. This is due to re-entry in the AV node or an accessory pathway (e.g. Wolff–Parkinson–White).

Ventricular fibrillation

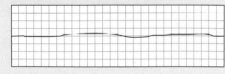

This occurs after the five QRS complexes. There are no QRS complexes, the baseline wanders, and there is no regularity to the ECG. The ventricular wall is fibrillating and there is no organized contraction. Immediate intervention is necessary as death is imminent.

Asystole

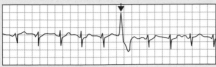

There is an absence of any heart contraction and there are no complexes in the ECG. The baseline is seen to wander slightly, but is essentially flat.

Other abnormalities

The following also affect the electrocardiogram:

- Digoxin – ST depression, T wave inversion.
- Hyperkalaemia – tall T waves, wide QRS complexes, absent P waves.
- Hypokalaemia – prolonged QT interval, small T waves, U waves (wave after T wave).
- Hypercalcaemia – short QT interval.
- Hypocalcaemia – long QT interval.

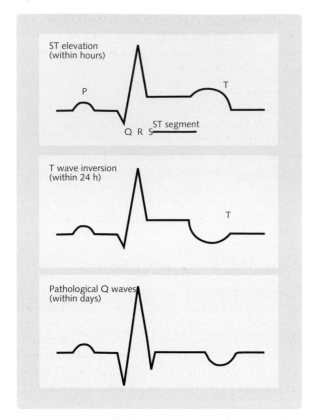

Fig. 9.12 ST elevation, T wave inversion, and Q waves after a myocardial infarction. Abnormal Q waves result from an electrode over an area of full thickness infarction.

Echocardiography

Echocardiography is increasingly used as a diagnostic technique. The echoes of ultrasound waves are used to study the heart and its function. As the ultrasound beam travels through the body, echoes are produced at tissue interfaces and are reflected back. Echoes from tissues furthest from the transmitter take longest to return. In this way, a picture is built up. Fluid generally shows up as black, tissues show up as white. Colour is used to indicate blood flow on machines that combine echocardiography with Doppler ultrasonography (see below).

Advantages of echocardiography for cardiovascular investigation include:

- Non-invasive, painless, and harmless.
- Can be used to study the motion of the heart and valves.
- Can be used to measure velocity of blood (using the Doppler shift phenomenon) and to

estimate stenosis severity from acceleration of blood through a lesion.
- Can be used to assess left ventricular function and size for a diagnosis of heart failure.

Disadvantages include the fact that the ribs and lungs do not allow ultrasound to pass through them, so special sites (or windows) must be used. Most imaging is still done through the anterior chest wall, but, when necessary, an oesophageal probe can be used for transoesophageal (TOE) imaging.

Echocardiography is used to investigate:

- Valvular disease.
- Pericardial effusion.
- Aneurysms.
- Left ventricular size for a diagnosis of heart failure.

Doppler ultrasonography

This is used to measure flow in peripheral vessels to provide information about the arteries (e.g. in peripheral vascular disease) and the veins (e.g. in suspected deep venous thrombosis). It uses ultrasound, in a similar way to that in echocardiography, to map out the vessel – highlighting any stenosis.

Red blood cells move relative to the ultrasound beam. They create a Doppler shift, which is a change in the frequency of the ultrasound echo that returns to the transducer. The shift in frequency is directly proportional to the velocity of the blood.

Colour can be used to differentiate blood flowing towards the probe from blood flowing away. It is commonly used to assess peripheral vessel function before a site is selected for angiography.

Doppler can also be used to calculate the ankle–brachial pressure index (ABPI). The Doppler derived systolic pressure from one of the foot pulses in the ankle (usually the dorsalis pedis) is divided into the Doppler derived systolic pressure in the brachial artery. This ratio provides useful information about the severity of peripheral vascular disease:

- ABPI >1 indicates normal vessel calibre (the blood pressure in the feet may be slightly higher than in the arms due to the effect of gravity).
- ABPI <0.7 indicates a degree of peripheral vascular disease (the blood pressure in the feet

is less than that in the arm due to atheroma formation or diabetic vessel changes).
- ABPI <0.3 indicates critical ischaemia (the blood pressure in the feet is so low it is likely the patient will be experiencing symptoms of ischaemia when resting).

Cardiac catheterization

Originally performed to directly measure the pressures in the right heart, left ventricle, aorta and pulmonary artery in patients with valvular disease, catheterization is now primarily used for angiography (see below). Echocardiography is now the method of choice to assess valvular function.

A thin radio-opaque catheter is introduced into the circulation, usually via the groin or wrist, and is then advanced towards the heart using fluoroscopy. The right heart is reached through a peripheral vein by threading the catheter through the right atrium, the right ventricle and into the pulmonary arteries. The left heart is reached by a catheter entered through a peripheral artery and advanced through the aorta and the aortic valve into the left ventricle.

To produce an angiogram, the catheter is used to inject a radio-opaque contrast medium into the heart or vessels. Angiograms are especially useful for viewing the coronary arteries for any stenosis. They are often performed before angioplasty or coronary artery bypass graft operations. Peripheral arteries can also be viewed with a similar process with the catheter being guided to the arterial tree to be viewed.

If right heart catheterization is performed, blood samples can also be taken to measure levels of local metabolites in the heart. Congenital shunts can be estimated from measurements of oxygen saturation at different sites in the heart.

Nuclear cardiology

Nuclear cardiology is used to look at myocardial function, especially in ischaemia. It uses radioisotopes, which emit radioactive particles that can be detected by gamma-camera.

Different radioisotopes have different affinities for various tissues; for example, thallium-201 is taken up by healthy myocardium, but not by ischaemic myocardium, thereby mapping the ischaemic area as a cold spot.

The technique can be used for subjects at rest and during exercise, but is usually used as an alternative for patients who are unable to perform an exercise tolerance test.

- Myocardial perfusion scan – this is done before and after exercise to detect ischaemia and infarction using a technetium tracer bound to tetrofosmin.
- Radionuclide ventriculography – uses blood labelled with technetium-99m to assess ventricular structure and function. Ventricular diastolic and systolic volumes are measured, which can be used to calculate the ejection fraction.

Pulmonary investigation

The pulmonary circulation can be investigated using ventilation/perfusion (V/Q) tests, which check for mismatches between air entry and the supply of blood to the alveoli (fully described in *Crash Course: Respiratory System*). More invasive tests include pulmonary angiography (usually imaged by CT scan), particularly when pulmonary emboli are suspected.

Biochemical markers of myocardial damage

Cellular enzymes and other intracellular proteins are released by necrotic tissue. Testing for the proteins specifically released from cardiac tissues can be a useful aid in confirming myocardial infarction (Fig. 9.13). The enzymes tested for include creatine kinase (CK), aspartate aminotransferase (AST), and lactate dehydrogenase (LDH), although these tests have largely been replaced by measurement of troponin T (Tn-T) or troponin I (Tn-I).

Troponins

Troponins are regulatory proteins on thin filaments which leak from damaged myocytes, peaking 12–24 hours after myocardial injury but frequently remaining elevated for over a week (and hence have replaced lactate dehydrogenase for the retrospective diagnosis of myocardial infarction). Elevated plasma Tn-T (and Tn-I) is both very sensitive and very specific for cardiac damage, but episodes of reversible ischaemia and renal failure may also elevate plasma troponin levels. The normal range of troponin varies significantly depending on the specific type of assay used.

Fig. 9.13 Schematic profile of the release of cardiac enzymes and markers. (Courtesy of Newby D E, Grubb N R. Cardiology: an illustrated colour text. Edinburgh: Elsevier, 2005.)

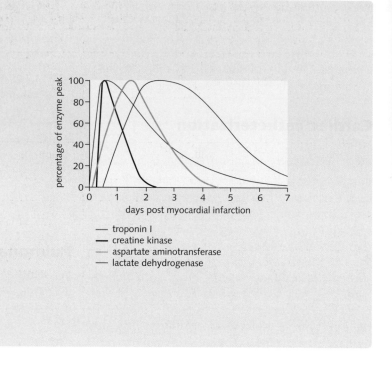

days post myocardial infarction

— troponin I
— creatine kinase
— aspartate aminotransferase
— lactate dehydrogenase

Creatine kinase

Creatine kinase peaks within 24 hours of infarction, and it returns to normal within 2 days. It is also produced by skeletal muscle and brain, so the isoenzyme specific to myocardium (CK-MB) is also sometimes measured. The level of enzyme released directly relates to the size of the infarction.

Creatine kinase levels can also be increased as a result of an intramuscular injection or the patient falling.

This enzyme is usually used to confirm a diagnosis of myocardial infarction.

Aspartate aminotransferase

Aspartate aminotransferase peaks after 1–2 days, and it returns to normal within 3 days. It is also produced from liver, kidney, lungs, and red blood cells.

Lactate dehydrogenase

Lactate dehydrogenase peaks after 2–3 days, and it stays high for 1 week. It is also released from skeletal muscle, liver, and red blood cells. LDH-1 – also known as hydroxybutyrate dehydrogenase (HBD) –

is the most cardiospecific of the five isoenzymes of lactate dehydrogenase. Lactate dehydrogenase is often used for a retrospective diagnosis of myocardial infarction.

ROUTINE INVESTIGATIONS

Haematology

Fig. 9.14 outlines the tests that can be performed when assessing haematological problems in the cardiovascular system.

Clinical chemistry

Frequently an abnormality in one investigation is not diagnostic of a condition. You must look at various factors to reach a definite diagnosis. For example, a raised ESR and white cell count may indicate infection, but this can only be proved by a positive culture or serological test.

Normal values for clinical haematology			
Component	Normal range	Change from normal	Reason
Haemoglobin	Male: 13–17 g/dL	High	Polycythaemia
	Female: 12–15 g/dL	Low	Anaemia
Red blood cells	Male: $4.4–5.8 \times 10^{12}$/L	High	Polycythaemia
	Female: $4.0–5.2 \times 10^{12}$/L	Low	Anaemia
White blood cells	$4–10 \times 10^9$/L	High	Infection, trauma, haemorrhage, inflammation, infarction
		Low	Infection, corticosteroid therapy
Platelet count	$150–400 \times 10^9$/L	High	Thrombocythaemia
		Low	Thrombocytopenia
Erythrocyte sedimentation rate (ESR)	Male: < (age in years)/2 Female: < (age in years + 10)/2	High: non-specific indication of disease	Myocardial infarction, vasculitis, systemic lupus erythematosus, rheumatoid arthritis, malignancy

Fig. 9.14 Normal values for clinical haematology.

Fig. 9.15 outlines the clinical chemistry tests that can be performed when assessing the cardiovascular system. Much biochemical data cannot be looked at individually (e.g. in dehydration there will probably be an increased concentration of sodium, potassium, chloride, etc.). Usually these tests are performed using blood, but urine can also be tested (e.g. for protein, glucose).

Microbiology

Any sample of the body can be sent for microscopy, cell culture and sensitivity testing. The microbiology department will attempt to grow any microorganisms present (culture) and determine what antibiotics can be used in treatment (sensitivity).

Viral serology may help to diagnose acute myocarditis (e.g. coxsackievirus). Samples sent are usually blood or sputum. Blood is indicated for suspected cases of infective endocarditis (e.g. *Streptococcus viridans*) and rheumatic fever (e.g. *Streptococcus pyogenes*). Sputum is indicated for suspected cases of tuberculosis (*Mycobacterium tuberculosis*).

Histopathology

Usually, samples sent for histopathological diagnosis are biopsies of the lesion. It is most commonly used for the following:

- Vasculitis – polyarteritis nodosa, Wegener's granulomatosis and Takayasu's arteritis.
- Cardiac tumours – atrial myxoma.
- Vascular tumours – haemangiomas.

IMAGING OF THE CARDIOVASCULAR SYSTEM

Radiography

Plain radiography

Examples of plain chest radiographs are shown in Figs 9.16–9.19.

Fig. 9.16 shows a normal posteroanterior (PA) chest radiograph. The width of the heart shadow is less than half of the transthoracic diameter. Note that it is only possible to comment on the heart size on the PA radiograph and not on an anteroposterior (AP) view.

A normal lateral chest radiograph is shown in Fig. 9.17. This is a useful view, especially if an abnormality is seen on the PA chest radiograph. It helps to localize any lesions. For example, left atrial enlargement is seen as a posterior projection indenting the oesophagus. Fig. 9.18 shows an aneurysm of the left ventricle. Fig. 9.19 shows heart failure and pulmonary oedema.

Normal values in clinical chemistry			
Substance analysed	Normal range	Change from normal	Causes
Urea	3.3–6.7 mmol/L	High	Renal failure
Creatinine	60–120 µmol/L	High	Renal failure
Electrolytes Na^+	135–145 mmol/L	High Low	Dehydration; hyperaldosteronism Diuretics; aldosterone deficiency; water excess
K^+	3.6–5.0 mmol/L	High or low	Can lead to arrhythmias
Cl^-	103–110 mmol/L	—	—
Ca^{2+}	2.2–2.6 mmol/L	High Low	Malignancy; thiazide diuretics; thyrotoxicosis Renal failure; blood transfusion
HCO_3^-	24–30 mmol/L	High Low	Metabolic/respiratory alkalosis Metabolic/respiratory acidosis
Glucose (fasting)	2.8–6.0 mmol/L	High	Impaired glucose tolerance
pO_2 (arterial)	11–15 kPa (85–105 mmHg)	Low	Respiratory failure Hyperventilation
pCO_2 (arterial)	4.5–6.0 kPa (35–46 mmHg)	Low High	Respiratory failure
Thyroid function TSH T_4 T_3	0.3–0.4 mU/L 9–26 pmol/L 3–8.8 pmol/L	High TSH, low T_4, T_3 Low TSH, high T_4, T_3	Hypothyroidism Hyperthyroidism
Cholesterol: total	<5.2 mmol/L	High	Hypercholesterolaemia (may be familial)
High-density lipoprotein	>1.2 mmol/L	Low	Predisposes to atherosclerosis
Low-density lipoprotein	<3.5 mmol/L	High	Hypercholesterolaemia (may be familial)
Triglyceride (fasting)	0.4–1.8 mmol/L	High	Hyperlipidaemia
Osmolality	280–295 mmol/L	High Low	Dehydration Water overload

Fig. 9.15 Normal values in clinical chemistry (T_3, tri-iodothyronine; T_4, thyroxine; TSH, thyroid stimulating hormone).

A 47-year-old female is admitted with sudden onset shortness of breath and pleuritic chest pain. A working diagnosis of pneumothorax is made, and an urgent chest x-ray is ordered. A good system for looking at radiographs is as follows:

- Name, age, and sex of patient.
- Date radiograph was taken.
- Is it AP (anteroposterior) or PA (posteroanterior)?
- Is it erect or supine?
- What is the penetration like (are the vertebral bodies just visible under the heart)?

- Is there any rotation (are the clavicles symmetrical)?
- Describe any abnormalities in:
  - Mediastinum.
  - Cardiac shadow.
  - Lung fields.
  - Bones, breasts and soft tissues.
  - Diaphragm.

After interpreting the chest x-ray, provide an opinion and formulate a management plan.

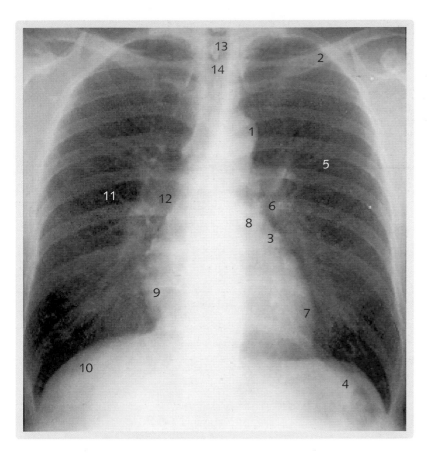

Fig. 9.16 Normal posteroanterior (PA) chest radiograph. 1, arch of aorta/aortic knuckle; 2, clavicle; 3, left atrial appendage; 4, left dome of diaphragm; 5, left lung; 6, left hilum; 7, left ventricular border; 8, pulmonary trunk; 9, right atrial border; 10, right dome of diaphragm; 11, right lung; 12, right hilum; 13, spine of vertebrae; 14, trachea. (Courtesy of Professor Dame M Turner-Warwick, Dr M Hodson, Professor B Corrin and Dr I Kerr.)

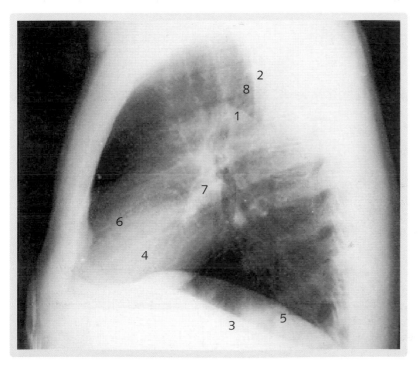

Fig. 9.17 Normal lateral chest radiograph. 1, aortic arch; 2, anterior borders of scapulae; 3, left dome of diaphragm; 4, left ventricle; 5, right dome of diaphragm; 6, right ventricle; 7, left atrium; 8, trachea. (Courtesy of Professor Dame M Turner-Warwick, Dr M Hodson, Professor B Corrin and Dr I Kerr.)

Fig. 9.18 Radiograph of an aneurysm of the left ventricle. This is a rare source of arterial embolism, which may occur some months after a myocardial infarct. Note the large heart shadow and how it occupies more than half of the transthoracic diameter. Contrast the normal appearance of the lung fields here with the congested fields in Fig. 9.19. (Courtesy of Professor J J F Belch, Mr P T McCollum, Mr P A Stonebridge and Professor W F Walker.)

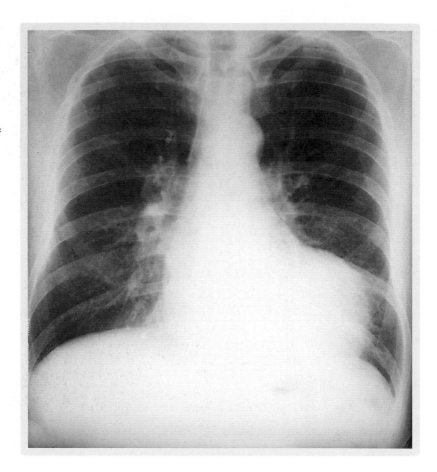

Fig. 9.19 Radiograph of the chest showing early pulmonary congestion. Note that the width of the heart shadow is greater than half the transthoracic diameter and that there are distended hila with increased lung markings. This indicates heart failure and pulmonary congestion. (Courtesy of Newby D E, Grubb N R. Cardiology: an illustrated colour text. Edinburgh: Elsevier, 2005.)

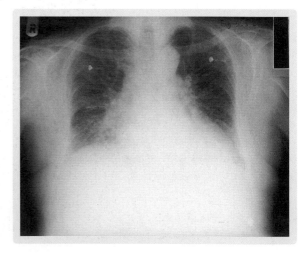

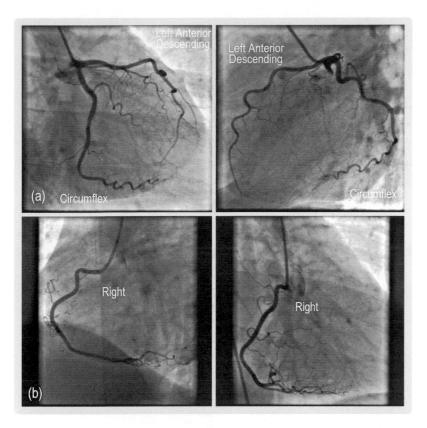

Fig 9.20 Coronary angiograms of normal left (A) and right (B) coronary arteries, each taken in two perpendicular views. (Courtesy of Newby D E, Grubb N R. Cardiology: an illustrated colour text. Edinburgh: Elsevier, 2005.)

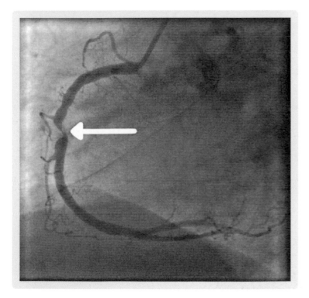

Fig 9.21 Coronary angiogram of a patient with a severe coronary stenosis (arrow). (Courtesy of Newby D E, Grubb N R. Cardiology: an illustrated colour text. Edinburgh: Elsevier, 2005.)

Angiography

Fig. 9.20 shows a normal angiogram of the left and right coronary arteries. Fig. 9.21 shows a definite stenosis which is likely to be symptomatic and requiring treatment.

Imaging of the pulmonary circulation

Fig. 9.22 shows examples of normal right and left pulmonary angiograms, while an example of pulmonary embolism of the right and left lobe is shown in Fig. 9.23. Computed tomography pulmonary angiograms (CTPA) are now frequently used to detect pulmonary embolism (Fig 9.24), as opposed to ventilation-perfusion (VQ) scans (Fig. 9.25).

Ultrasound

Echocardiography

A parasternal long axis view of a normal heart is shown in Fig. 9.26 while mitral stenosis is demonstrated in Fig. 9.27.

179

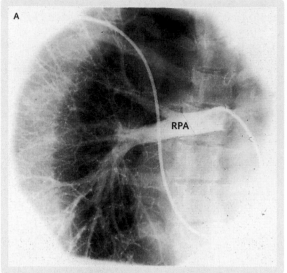

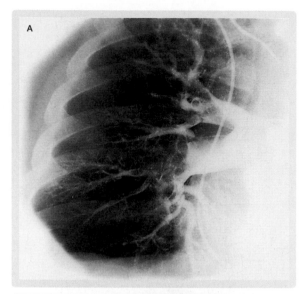

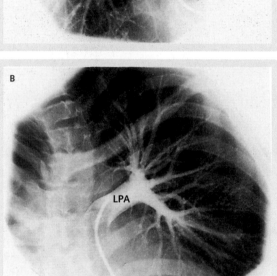

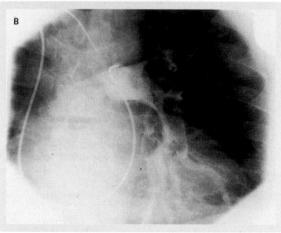

Fig. 9.23 Pulmonary angiograms showing pulmonary embolism of the right lung (A) and left lung (B). Contrast agent does not reach the distal part of the arterial tree, implying that there is some blockage. (Courtesy of Dr A Timmis and Dr S Brecker.)

Fig. 9.22 Normal right (A) and left (B) pulmonary angiograms. The contrast agent highlights the entire arterial tree from the right and left pulmonary arteries (LPA, left pulmonary artery; RPA, right pulmonary artery). (Courtesy of Dr A Timmis and Dr S Brecker.)

Tomography

Computerized tomography (CT)

An example of an aortic aneurysm is shown in Fig. 9.28.

This imaging modality enables precise measurement of the size of the aneurysm. The whole body is imaged as slices or sections using x-rays.

It can be used to produce a three-dimensional image, and it may also be used to perform angiography using radio-opaque contrast medium.

Magnetic resonance imaging (MRI)

MRI of the chest enables an accurate assessment to be made of the dimensions of the heart walls and lumen. Fig. 9.29 shows a normal coronal view of the chest, while Fig. 9.30 shows an extensive aortic dissection.

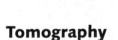

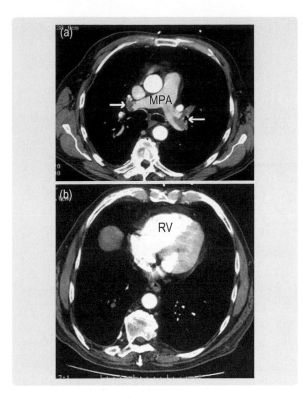

Fig 9.24 Computed tomography pulmonary angiogram showing (A) large central thromboemboli and (B) dilated right ventricle with bowing of the interventricular septum (MPA, main pulmonary artery; arrows, clot filling defects; RV, right ventricle). (Courtesy of Newby D E, Grubb N R. Cardiology: an illustrated colour text. Edinburgh: Elsevier, 2005.)

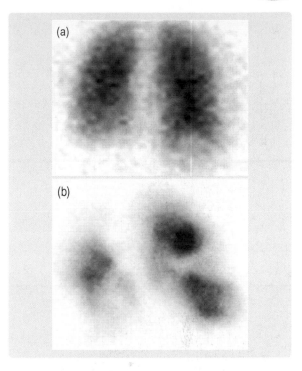

Fig 9.25 Radionuclide ventilation (a) and perfusion (b) scans showing normal ventilation but multiple perfusion defects characteristic of pulmonary thromboembolism. (Courtesy of Newby D E, Grubb N R. Cardiology: an illustrated colour text. Edinburgh: Elsevier, 2005.)

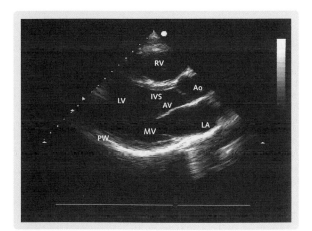

Fig. 9.26 Echocardiogram of the parasternal long axis view (diastolic frame) (Ao, aorta; AV, aortic valve; IVS, intraventricular septum; LA, left atrium; LV, left ventricle; MV, mitral valve; PW, posterior LV wall; RV, right ventricle). (Courtesy of Dr A Timmis and Dr S Brecker.)

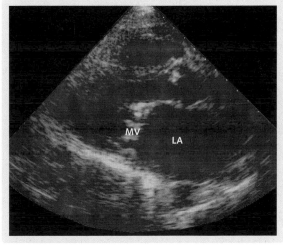

Fig. 9.27 Echocardiogram of mitral stenosis (long axis). The mitral valve (MV) leaflets are densely thickened and the left atrium (LA) is severely dilated. (Courtesy of Dr A Timmis and Dr S Brecker.)

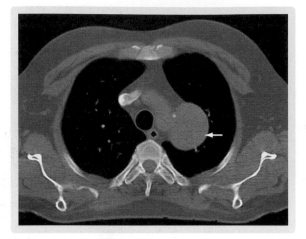

Fig. 9.28 CT of a thoracic aortic aneurysm. The scan shows a large aneurysm of the descending aortic arch (arrowed) arising just after the left subclavian branch. This is the typical location for dissecting aortic aneurysms although a dissection cannot be seen in this film. (Courtesy of Dr A Timmis and Dr S Brecker.)

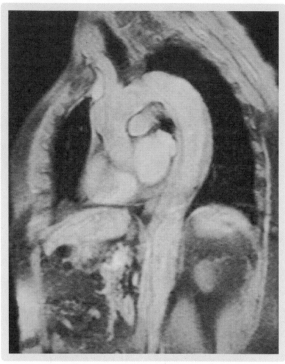

Fig. 9.30 Sagittal MRI scan showing extensive aortic dissection. Note how the descending aorta seems to have two lumens (double-barrelled). (Courtesy of Dr A Timmis and Dr S Brecker.)

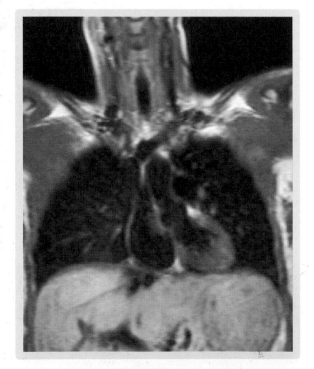

Fig. 9.29 Normal MRI coronal view of the chest. (Courtesy of Dr A Timmis and Dr S Brecker.)

MRI allows better visualization of soft tissue than CT. It is safer than CT as it does not involve harmful radiation. MRI may also be set to show moving blood, to produce an image similar to an angiogram. This has replaced conventional angiography for peripheral arteries, where MRI is available. Heart movement currently restricts the visualization of the coronary arteries to the large proximal vessels only.

The use of gadolinium as a contrast agent allows delineation of perfused myocardium during the first pass and of infarcted tissue 15–20 minutes later.

SELF-ASSESSMENT

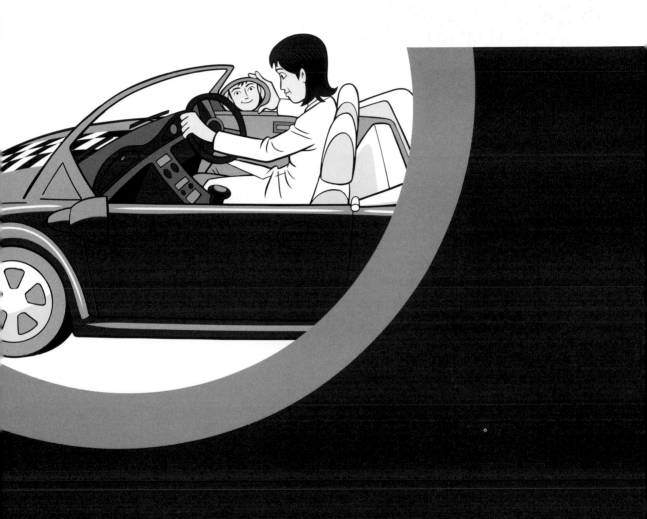

Multiple-choice questions

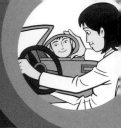

Indicate whether the following are true or false.

Chapter 1 – Overview of the cardiovascular system

1. **Functions of the cardiovascular system include:**
   a. Transport of nutrients.
   b. Hormonal control.
   c. Host defence.
   d. Temperature regulation.
   e. Reproduction.

2. **Concerning the organization of the cardiovascular system:**
   a. The pulmonary vein carries deoxygenated blood to the left atrium.
   b. The heart is an endocrine organ.
   c. The pulmonary vascular bed has a higher resistance than the systemic vasculature.
   d. The pressure is greater in the aorta than in the capillaries.
   e. The kidneys receive approximately 20% of the cardiac output.

Chapter 2 – Structure and function of the heart

3. **Concerning the anatomy of the mediastinum:**
   a. The thymus lies anteriorly in the mediastinum.
   b. The apex of the pericardium is fused with the central tendon of the diaphragm.
   c. The diaphragmatic surface of the heart is constructed mainly from the left ventricle.
   d. The apex of the heart is formed by the left ventricle and is posterior to the 5th intercostal space.
   e. There are four pulmonary veins.

4. **Concerning the anatomy of the internal structures of the heart:**
   a. The mitral valve has three cusps and lies between the left atrium and left ventricle.
   b. There are two left and one right coronary arteries.
   c. The pulmonary valve is a semilunar valve.
   d. The three arteries supplying the sinoatrial node are branches of the right coronary artery.
   e. The coronary veins eventually drain into the left atrium.

5. **Concerning the embryological development of the heart:**
   a. The heart only starts developing at 6 weeks' gestation.
   b. The atria are separated by the septum spurium.
   c. The truncus arteriosus rotates to align itself with the ventricles.
   d. The ventricular septum has a membranous part superior to a muscular section.
   e. The left atrium initially starts with only one pulmonary vein.

6. **Concerning the structure of the valves:**
   a. They are avascular.
   b. Papillary muscles are required for atrioventricular valve function.
   c. The aortic valve receives its nutrients from the lumen.
   d. The tricuspid valve is the valve most commonly affected by rheumatic fever.
   e. The pulmonary valve is stenosed in tetralogy of Fallot.

7. **In cardiac myocytes:**
   a. Myocyte resting potential is –90 mV.
   b. Positive inotropes act by reducing intracellular Ca^{2+}.
   c. Gap junctions hold myocytes together at branch points.
   d. Nodal, Purkinje fibre and contractile (work) cells are all myocytes.
   e. The pacemaker potential decays partly due to inward leakage of Na^+.

8. **The normal action potential:**
   a. Is dependent on cytoplasmic and extracellular Na^+ and K^+ ionic concentration differences.
   b. The resting myocyte membrane is most permeable to K^+.
   c. In nodal cells, Na^+ is responsible for a fast upstroke.
   d. The Nernst equation predicts ionic membrane permeability.
   e. The fast upstroke in contractile cells is mediated by K^+.

9. **Regarding excitation–contraction coupling:**

   a. Cytoplasmic Ca^{2+} influx couples excitation and contraction.
   b. The increased force of contraction associated with an increased heart rate is known as the Treppe effect.
   c. Produces tension proportional to the level of Ca^{2+}.
   d. Changes in contractility are mediated by changes in Ca^{2+} concentration.
   e. Positive chronotropes increase the strength of contraction.

10. **In the cardiac cycle:**

    a. The ventricles fill during diastole.
    b. Myocardial perfusion occurs during diastole.
    c. Atrial contraction is essential for ventricular filling.
    d. The first heart sound occurs at the start of systole.
    e. The mitral valve opens when left atrial pressure is greater than left ventricular pressure.

11. **The following are true for Starling's law:**

    a. The force of contraction is inversely proportional to the initial length of the cardiac muscle fibre.
    b. The law is only true for isolated heart–lung preparations.
    c. The law means that the stroke volume is proportional to end-diastolic volume unless the contractility or vascular resistance changes.
    d. As a consequence of the law, factors that reduce cardiac filling will increase contractility.
    e. The law is dependent on the integrity of the cardiac stretch receptors.

12. **In the normal heart:**

    a. Cardiac output is the product of heart rate and end-diastolic volume.
    b. Contractility is defined as the force of contraction for a given fibre length.
    c. End-diastolic volume and end-diastolic pressure are closely related.
    d. The Starling curve peaks and turns down due to overstretch of individual myocytes.
    e. Total peripheral resistance is defined as arterial pressure divided by cardiac output.

13. **In the electrocardiogram:**

    a. Atrial repolarization is represented by the t wave.
    b. The R–R interval can be used to calculate the ventricular rate.
    c. The R wave coincides with depolarization of the apex.
    d. A P–R interval of 120 ms may be found in a normal healthy adult.
    e. The first heart sound coincides with the P wave.

Chapter 3 – Structure and function of the vessels

14. **Concerning the classification of vessels:**

    a. The presence of fibrous tissue in arteries decreases with distance from the heart.
    b. Fluid and metabolites return to the heart through veins and lymphatic vessels.
    c. Vessels are supplied exclusively from blood within the lumen.
    d. The vasculature consists of conductance, resistance and capacitance vessels.
    e. The diameter of the aorta is approximately 5 mm.

15. **Concerning the anatomy of the aorta:**

    a. The brachial artery is a branch of the aorta.
    b. The wall of the aorta is approximately 2 mm thick.
    c. The brachiocephalic trunk, left common carotid and left subclavian all branch off in the thorax.
    d. The first branch of the aorta is the brachiocephalic trunk.
    e. The renal arteries branch off the aorta before its bifurcation.

16. **Concerning the arteries of the abdomen:**

    a. The coeliac trunk supplies the mid-gut structures.
    b. The right gastric artery is a branch of the coeliac trunk.
    c. The sigmoid colon is supplied by the sigmoid arteries.
    d. The majority of the small intestine is supplied by the superior mesenteric artery.
    e. The right gastric artery supplies the greater curvature of the stomach.

17. **Concerning the arteries of the head and neck:**

    a. The circle of Willis is not a complete circle.
    b. The ophthalmic artery is a division of the internal carotid artery.
    c. The external jugular vein joins the internal jugular vein on its return to the heart.
    d. The facial artery is a branch of the internal carotid artery.
    e. The veins of the head and neck eventually drain into the superior vena cava.

18. **At birth:**

    a. Pulmonary vasculature resistance falls rapidly.
    b. After birth, the atrial pressures are equal.
    c. Prostaglandins are involved in maintaining the patency of the ductus venosus.
    d. The umbilical cord should be clamped within 3 seconds.
    e. The septum primum closes the foramen ovale.

19. **Regarding regulation of smooth muscle cell tension:**
    a. EDRF requires cGMP to produce relaxation.
    b. Adrenaline requires cAMP to produce vasodilatation.
    c. Sympathetic innervation of smooth muscle uses noradrenaline.
    d. Hypoxia produces relaxation through hyperpolarization of the membrane.
    e. Tension in smooth muscle requires as much energy to maintain as in skeletal muscle.

20. **The pressure wave created by ventricular ejection depends upon:**
    a. Stroke volume.
    b. Heart rate.
    c. Elasticity of the arterial wall.
    d. Peripheral vascular resistance.
    e. Blood volume.

21. **In the measurement of blood pressure:**
    a. Isolated systolic hypertension occurs frequently in the elderly.
    b. It is measured in mmH_2O.
    c. Mean arterial pressure is the most important determinant of organ perfusion.
    d. Blood pressure rises during sleep.
    e. Korotkoff I and V sounds are used.

22. **Flow through the vessels:**
    a. Varies with the pressure difference between one end and the other.
    b. Is directly proportional to the square of the radius.
    c. Increases directly with the length of the vessel.
    d. Varies inversely with the viscosity of the blood.
    e. Is directly proportional to the velocity of the blood.

23. **Concerning haemostasis and thrombosis:**
    a. Haemostasis is a static balance between production and degradation of clot.
    b. Clotting may be initiated by endothelial cell injury.
    c. Haemophilia is an X-linked condition which mainly affects males.
    d. Factor V Leiden is a common mutation resulting in a tendency to bleed.
    e. Thrombocythaemia promotes thrombus formation.

24. **Concerning the haemodynamics of veins:**
    a. Normal central venous pressure is 12–20 mmHg.
    b. Tension in the smooth muscle of veins is controlled by sympathetic nervous stimulation.
    c. Orthostasis causes a decrease in blood pressure.
    d. Rhythmic contraction of skeletal muscle in the legs results in a rise in central venous pressure.
    e. In the central veins, flow decreases during inspiration.

25. **Capillaries:**
    a. Contain, at any one time, 50% of the blood volume.
    b. Have a diameter that is about the same as that of a red blood cell.
    c. Have precapillary sphincters of smooth muscle.
    d. Allow lipid soluble substances to directly cross their walls.
    e. Control vascular resistance by constricting their walls.

26. **Concerning capillary transport mechanisms:**
    a. Hydrostatic pressure is the main determinant of fluid shift at the arterial end of the capillary.
    b. Hydrostatic pressure is typically 37 mmHg at the arterial end.
    c. Tension in the capillary is proportional to both pressure difference and radius.
    d. Fluid exchange is important for nutrient and metabolite exchange.
    e. Hypoproteinaemia results in an increase in osmotic pressure and subsequent oedema.

27. **Lymphatics:**
    a. Drain excess filtrate from the interstitium.
    b. Return lymph to the subclavian artery.
    c. Play a role in the immune response by transferring antigen to lymph nodes.
    d. Are the main transport of protein from the gut.
    e. Are very extensive in the brain.

Chapter 4 – control of the cardiovascular system

28. **Regarding regulation of blood flow:**
    a. Nitric oxide mediates the response to hypoxia.
    b. Autoregulation describes the regulation of blood flow in response to blood pressure changes.
    c. Hyperaemia is a pathological increase in blood flow.
    d. Increased sympathetic activity produces only vasoconstriction.
    e. Increased parasympathetic activity leads solely to vasodilatation.

29. **Regarding hormonal control:**
    a. Renin is released from stromal cells in the kidney.
    b. Brain natriuretic peptide is released from the ventricles in response to stretch.
    c. Vasopressin is released from the hypothalamus in response to osmolarity changes.
    d. Angiotensin I acts on smooth muscle to produce vasoconstriction.
    e. Aldosterone increases Na^+ and water retention.

30. **Myogenic autoregulation:**
    a. Keeps blood flow constant despite changes in mean arterial blood pressure.
    b. Is caused by contraction of smooth muscle induced by stretch.
    c. Keeps blood flow constant regardless of metabolic activity.
    d. Is dependent on neuronal innervation.
    e. Is unaffected by hypoxia.

31. **If blood pressure falls, reflex effects mediated by baroreceptors include:**
    a. Constriction of cerebral arterioles.
    b. Constriction of skeletal muscle arterioles.
    c. Constriction of veins.
    d. Decrease in ventilation.
    e. Increase in force of cardiac contraction.

32. **Concerning the distribution of cardiac output:**
    a. The heart receives approximately 10%.
    b. The brain can receive up to 30% when in deep concentration.
    c. Blood delivery to skeletal muscle increases during exercise.
    d. The high blood flow to the kidneys is as a result of high oxygen requirement.
    e. The skin has the highest blood flow per 100 g of any organ.

33. **Concerning hormonal control of the cardiovascular system:**
    a. Adrenaline is secreted from the adrenal cortex.
    b. Renin is converted to angiotensin I by angiotensinogen.
    c. ACE is predominately found in the vascular bed of the gastrointestinal tract.
    d. ADH is released when a rise in osmolarity is detected.
    e. Adrenaline causes vasodilatation in skeletal muscle, myocardium and the liver.

34. **Concerning the cardiovascular response to exercise:**
    a. Blood flow to skeletal muscle can increase by as much as 40 times normal.
    b. Cardiac output is increased.
    c. Training results in a thin-walled dilated ventricle.
    d. Blood flow to the skin increases to increase heat loss.
    e. Cardiac output increases because of the Starling mechanism.

Chapter 5 – The cardiovascular system in disease – diseases of the heart

35. **Risk factors for cardiovascular disease include:**
    a. Blood disorders such as haemophilia.
    b. Diabetes mellitus.
    c. Early menopause.
    d. Obesity.
    e. Thrombocythaemia.

36. **Concerning the treatment of angina:**
    a. An important treatment principle is slowing heart rate.
    b. Verapamil may cause a profound bradycardia.
    c. Ramipril is a Ca^{2+} channel blocker.
    d. Side effects of ACE inhibitors include worsening asthma, bradycardia and syncope.
    e. GTN is usually given sublingually in the acute situation.

37. **In myocardial infarction:**
    a. The vessel usually affected is the right coronary artery.
    b. Ventricular aneurysm may occur as an acute complication.
    c. It takes 120 minutes for irreversible injury to occur from the onset of ischaemia.
    d. Scar formation occurs after approximately 12 days.
    e. Subendocardial infarction usually occurs as a result of an acute plaque change.

38. **The following are recognized complications of myocardial infarction:**
    a. Sudden death.
    b. Aortic valve displacement.
    c. Cerebrovascular accident.
    d. Cirrhosis of the liver.
    e. Thrombosis: central or peripheral.

39. **The following are true of heart failure:**
    a. Reduced contractility reduces stroke volume for a given filling pressure.
    b. Renal retention of K^+ occurs.
    c. Pathologically, the chamber is thin-walled and dilated.
    d. Shortness of breath is more marked on standing.
    e. ACE inhibitors have been shown to prolong life in heart failure.

40. Concerning atrial fibrillation:

a. Alcohol may predispose to this arrhythmia.
b. The atrial component of ventricular filling is lost.
c. The pulse is irregular in rate, but regular in volume.
d. There are no P waves present on the electrocardiogram.
e. Treatment may include DC cardioversion.

41. A ventricular rather than a supraventricular tachycardia is suggested by:

a. A ventricular rate of >160 beats per minute.
b. Termination of arrhythmia with carotid sinus pressure.
c. The presence of irregular canon A waves.
d. The presence of cardiac failure.
e. QRS complexes >120 ms on an electrocardiogram.

42. Regarding cardiac rhythms:

a. Supraventricular rhythms all originate in the atrioventricular node.
b. A normal rate is between 40 and 120 beats per minute.
c. Sinus arrhythmia is normal.
d. Tachycardia or atrial fibrillation frequently occur in Wolff–Parkinson–White syndrome.
e. The PR interval is increased with first degree heart block.

43. Amiodarone may cause:

a. Pulmonary alveolitis.
b. Liver damage.
c. Constipation.
d. Asthma.
e. Thyroid disorders.

44. Angina:

a. Is caused by ischaemic myocardium.
b. Is never life-threatening.
c. May be caused by atheromatous changes.
d. Treatment involves increasing cardiac output.
e. Can be treated with verapamil.

45. Myocardial infarction:

a. Immediately results in ST elevation.
b. May lead to ventricular rupture and cardiac tamponade.
c. Commonly results from platelet aggregation or thrombosis.
d. May begin as a subendocardial infarction, which progresses to become transmural.
e. Myocyte loss may continue even after reperfusion.

46. Regarding the pericardium:

a. It normally contains 200 mL of fluid.
b. Pericardial effusions can be serous, serosanguineous or chylous.
c. Cardiac tamponade is a medical emergency.
d. Pericarditis is a recognized complication of rheumatoid arthritis.
e. Serous effusions result from pericardial infection.

47. Syncope:

a. May be caused by coughing.
b. May be a sign of an intracardiac tumour.
c. Associated with facial flushing suggests an arrhythmia.
d. Is commonly caused by vasovagal attack.
e. May be caused by excessive exercise in patients with mitral regurgitation.

48. Cardiomyopathy:

a. The term 'cardiomyopathy' implies a known aetiology.
b. Is classified as restrictive, hypertrophic or dilated.
c. Restrictive cardiomyopathy is associated with an increase in ventricular mass.
d. Excessive catecholamine levels may cause a dilated cardiomyopathy.
e. Dilated cardiomyopathy may lead to heart failure, thromboembolism, and arrhythmia.

49. Endocarditis:

a. Infective endocarditis is classified according to the infective organism.
b. May occur after dental treatment.
c. Is more common in IV drug users.
d. May arise without an infection.
e. Can result in peripheral emboli.

50. In rheumatic fever:

a. There is often a preceding group A β-haemolytic streptococcal infection.
b. Skin rash may occur, especially in children.
c. There is a raised erythrocyte sedimentation rate (ESR).
d. Small joint rather than large joint pain is typical.
e. Large vegetations are present on the valves.

51. Coronary artery bypass grafting:

a. Is more effective than medical therapy at prolonging life in patients with angina.
b. Has a reduced risk of re-stenosis when compared with that of angioplasty.
c. Commonly uses grafts made from artificial substances.
d. Is routinely offered to all patients.
e. Results in a reduced requirement for anti-anginal drugs.

52. Concerning cardiac tumours:

a. Metastatic tumours are more common than primary.
b. Pulmonary embolism occurs in some patients with myxomas.
c. Myxomas typically arise is the right atrium.
d. Echocardiography is useful for identifying the location and shape of the tumour.
e. They may mimic endocarditis with valve dysfunction and emboli.

53. Concerning left-to-right congenital shunts:

a. Atrial septal defects are the most common congenital defect.
b. Most ventricular septal defects close spontaneously within the first two years of life.
c. A patent ductus arteriosus is associated with a continuous machinery murmur.
d. Atrial septal defect is associated with a soft diastolic murmur.
e. Atrial-ventricular septal defect is associated with Down syndrome.

54. Obstructive congenital defects:

a. Coarctation of the aorta usually occurs around the area of the ductus arteriosus.
b. Coarctation of the aorta is associated with a ventricular septal defect and a bicuspid aortic valve.
c. Weak radial pulses are a feature of coarctation of the aorta.
d. Pulmonary stenosis represents 20% of cardiac defects.
e. Heart failure, syncope and chest pain are all features of tricuspid stenosis.

55. Concerning right-to-left congenital shunts:

a. Transposition of the great arteries occurs from failure of the truncocanal septum to spiral.
b. Eisenmenger's syndrome occurs due to a low pressure developing in the pulmonary vasculature.
c. Eisenmenger's syndrome is easily treatable with drug therapy.
d. Pulmonary stenosis and left ventricular hypertrophy are both features of tetralogy of Fallot.
e. Clubbing may be seen.

56. The following are true of diseases affecting the pericardium:

a. Haemopericardium may occur secondary to a deep vein thrombosis.
b. Cardiac tamponade requires a minimum of 500 mL in the pericardial space.
c. Viral pericarditis causes a fibrous exudate.
d. Pericarditis frequently occurs in rheumatic fever.
e. Kussmaul's sign is a feature of cardiac tamponade.

57. Concerning myocarditis:

a. It may be caused by viruses, bacteria, protozoa and fungi.
b. Dilatation occurs in the ventricles only.
c. It predisposes to thrombosis.
d. The clinical picture may be mistaken for myocardial infarction.
e. It may be easily treated with β-blockers.

Chapter 6 – The cardiovascular system in disease – diseases of the vessels

58. Regarding shock:

a. Results solely from acute blood loss.
b. Is compensated for by Na^+ and water retention.
c. Should always be treated with adrenaline.
d. Only results in a fall in blood pressure with loss of >30% of blood volume.
e. Peripheral vasoconstriction is a sign of hypovolaemic shock.

59. Pathogenesis of atheroma is thought to:

a. Involve platelets.
b. Involve smooth muscle cells.
c. Involve macrophages.
d. Involve endothelial cell damage.
e. Involve multiple cytokines.

60. In the treatment of hypertension:

a. α-Adrenoreceptor agonists are beneficial.
b. Centrally acting drugs include methyldopa.
c. Cyanide poisoning may result from administration of inorganic nitrates.
d. Potassium channel agonists hyperpolarize smooth muscle cells, producing vasodilatation.
e. Angiotensin II receptor antagonists are associated with dry cough.

61. In relation to lipid metabolism:

a. Apolipoproteins act as docking proteins for lipoproteins.
b. Oxidized low-density lipoprotein (LDL) is chemotactic for macrophages.
c. Type I hyperlipidaemia is treated by diet alone.
d. Statins are a useful treatment for hypertrygliceridaemia (type IV).
e. Resins affect lipid metabolism in adipose tissue.

62. In haemorrhagic shock there is:

a. Decreased urinary output.
b. Sweating.
c. Thirst.
d. Increased total peripheral resistance.
e. Bradycardia.

63. Concerning hyperlipidaemia:

a. Type II hyperlipidaemia typically raises cholesterol.
b. Raised high-density lipoprotein (HDL) levels are a known risk factor for coronary heart disease.
c. Hypercholesterolaemia is a common cause of pancreatitis.
d. Diabetes mellitus is associated with some hyperlipidaemias.
e. Pravastatin is an ion-exchange resin that can be used to lower cholesterol levels in the blood.

64. Hypertension:

a. Is defined by the World Health Organization as blood pressure above 140 mmHg systolic or 90 mmHg diastolic in any patient.
b. Results exclusively from arteriolar smooth muscle contraction.
c. Can be treated safely in the elderly with an angiotensin-converting enzyme (ACE) inhibitor.
d. Control of blood pressure has no effect on cardiovascular morbidity.
e. Many elderly patients also suffer from postural hypotension, so care must be taken in prescribing treatment.

65. Concerning dissecting aortic aneurysms:

a. Aortic regurgitation is common.
b. Pain often radiates to the back.
c. It is essential to identify the point of re-entry so that surgery can be successful.
d. Computerized tomography of the thorax is helpful in the diagnosis.
e. May be caused by syphilis.

66. Concerning the vasculitides:

a. Giant cell arteritis often presents with headaches, temporal pain and polymyalgia.
b. Kawasaki disease usually occurs in children, and it can cause coronary aneurysms.
c. Polyarteritis nodosa typically affects large arteries.
d. Wegener's granulomatosis typically involves the lungs and kidneys.
e. Thromboangiitis obliterans usually affects non-smokers.

67. Concerning haemangiomas:

a. They more commonly affect children.
b. Granuloma pyogenicum is a type of capillary haemangioma that occurs in a pregnant woman.
c. They may present as strawberry naevi on the face of infants.
d. Capillary haemangiomas are found only in the skin.
e. They are benign tumours of blood vessels.

68. In deep vein thrombosis:

a. Many patients have ankle oedema.
b. Pulmonary embolism can result in pyrexia.
c. Doppler ultrasonography can be useful.
d. Malignancy should be suspected if no obvious predisposing factor can be found.
e. Lifelong treatment should always be given.

69. The following may be signs of shock:

a. Hypotension.
b. Bradycardia.
c. A rise in pulse pressure.
d. Increased urine output.
e. Warm, flushed skin.

70. In the immediate response to haemorrhage:

a. Total peripheral resistance increases.
b. Erythropoietin production increases.
c. Renin production is increased.
d. There is stimulation of both baroreceptors and chemoreceptors.
e. Increased angiotensin II levels promote thirst.

71. Concerning abdominal aortic aneurysm:

a. It is a 'saccular' aneurysm.
b. Their prevalence is estimated to be approximately 3% in men over 50 years.
c. Hypertension increases the risk of rupture.
d. Operative mortality in the emergency situation is approximately 5%.
e. The aneurysm is usually above the level of the renal arteries.

72. Concerning aneurysms:

a. These are abnormal, localized, temporary dilatations.
b. They are confined exclusively to arteries.
c. They may be caused by Chlamydia.
d. Most commonly occur in the abdominal aorta.
e. A false aneurysm is one which is sometimes normal.

73. In dissecting aortic aneurysms:

a. The pulses of the upper limbs may be asymmetrical.
b. The tear occurs in the intima.
c. Type A aneurysms occur in the ascending part of the thoracic aorta.
d. Type B aneurysms are treated surgically.
e. Haemopericardium is a potential complication.

74. Congenital abnormalities of the vessels:

a. Include atrial septal defect.
b. Vascular rings may form around the oesophagus leading to difficulty swallowing.
c. Secondary lymphoedema occurs secondary to hypoplasia of the lymphatic system.
d. An arteriovenous fistula is an abnormal communication between an artery and a vein.
e. The kidney may occasionally have a double renal supply.

191

75. Concerning berry aneurysms:

a. These are a common cause of headache.
b. When they bleed, they do so into the subdural space.
c. They are more likely to rupture in young women.
d. They always occur in the same place.
e. Smoking is a risk factor for rupture.

76. Concerning varicose veins:

a. These are dilated, tortuous deep veins.
b. Immobility and lying flat are strong risk factors.
c. They often occur as a sequelae of deep vein thrombosis.
d. They must always be treated to prevent complications.
e. Histologically, the wall becomes thickened.

77. Concerning deep vein thrombosis:

a. Recent surgery is a risk factor.
b. They can be asymptomatic.
c. Thrombophlebitis migrans is indicative of underlying malignancy.
d. Initial treatment is with warfarin.
e. Most commonly occur in the calves.

78. In peripheral vascular disease:

a. The pain of claudication is sharp and exacerbated by rest.
b. Patients should receive aspirin.
c. Smoking is protective against disease.
d. β-Blockers are the anti-hypertensive of choice.
e. Patients are at an increased risk of ischaemic heart disease.

79. Peripheral vascular disease:

a. Most commonly affects the superficial femoral artery.
b. Absence of a foot pulse is always abnormal.
c. May cause ulcers.
d. Is more common in the elderly.
e. Statins are contraindicated.

Chapter 7 – Common presentations of cardiovascular disease

80. Cardiovascular presenting complaints may be:

a. Syncope.
b. Visual impairment.
c. Nausea and vomiting.
d. Shortness of breath at night.
e. Neurological defects.

81. Causes of central chest pain include:

a. Dissecting aortic aneurysm.
b. Pulmonary embolism.
c. Pneumothorax.
d. Oesophagitis.
e. Pericarditis.

82. In cardiac arrest:

a. Ventricular fibrillation should be treated with immediate defibrillation.
b. All patients should receive adrenaline.
c. All patients should receive atropine.
d. Tension pneumothorax is a potentially reversible cause.
e. Is defined by an absent cardiac output.

Chapter 8 – History and examination

83. The following pulse types are associated with these diseases:

a. Pulsus alternans – left ventricular disease.
b. Slow rising pulse – aortic stenosis.
c. Collapsing pulse – hypotension.
d. Pulsus paradoxus – cardiac tamponade.
e. Pulsus bisferiens – pulmonary hypertension.

84. Classic abnormalities of the jugular venous pulse include:

a. Absent 'a' waves in atrial fibrillation.
b. Giant 'a' waves in tricuspid regurgitation.
c. Large 'v' waves in pulmonary regurgitation.
d. A slow 'y' descent in tricuspid stenosis.
e. A raised jugular venous pressure on inspiration (Kussmaul's sign) with pericardial tamponade.

85. Correct findings on auscultation include:

a. The first heart sound immediately follows the carotid pulse upstroke.
b. Expiration causes physiological splitting of the second heart sound.
c. A loud opening snap in diastole suggests mitral valve disease.
d. The fourth heart sound, if present, coincides with atrial systole.
e. A mid-diastolic click indicates mitral valve prolapse.

86. The following heart sounds have these inferences:

a. Splitting of the second heart sound – left bundle branch block.
b. Pansystolic murmur – mitral regurgitation.
c. Ejection systolic – pulmonary stenosis.
d. Mid-diastolic murmur – tricuspid stenosis.
e. Continuous murmur – aortic stenosis and regurgitation.

87. In inspiration:

a. The murmur of ventricular septal defect gets louder.
b. Reverse splitting of the second heart sound occurs in pulmonary hypertension.
c. Blood pressure falls with constrictive pericarditis.
d. The heart rate is unaffected in the young.
e. Pulmonary venous flow increases.

88. The following are features of peripheral vascular disease:

a. Warm, well-perfused skin.
b. Absent foot pulses.
c. Ulceration on the heel of the foot.
d. Nausea and vomiting.
e. Shiny, hairless skin.

89. The following are important features of a cardiovascular history:

a. Smoking status.
b. Family history of ischaemic heart disease.
c. Herbal remedies taken, e.g. St John's wort.
d. Recent thirst and excessive urination.
e. History of liver cirrhosis.

90. The following are causes of clubbing:

a. Infective endocarditis.
b. Atrial septal defect.
c. Myocardial infarction.
d. Tetralogy of Fallot.
e. Eisenmenger's syndrome.

91. Concerning cardiac murmurs and auscultation:

a. Aortic stenosis is an ejection systolic murmur.
b. Mitral regurgitation is best heard at the apex.
c. Aortic regurgitation frequently radiates to the carotids.
d. Patent ductus arteriosus causes a continuous murmur.
e. Mitral stenosis gets quieter during exercise.

92. On examination of the abdomen:

a. A midline expansile mass is suggestive of an abdominal aortic aneurysm.
b. An enlarged kidney indicates congestive cardiac failure.
c. A pulsatile liver indicates mitral regurgitation.
d. Venous blood flow away from the umbilicus is suggestive of superior vena cava obstruction.
e. Ascites may occur as the result of heart failure.

Chapter 9 – Investigations and imaging

93. Effective imaging techniques for diagnosing specific disease include:

a. Plain chest radiograph – pulmonary embolism.
b. Computerized tomography – aortic aneurysm.
c. Magnetic resonance imaging – myocardial hypertrophy.
d. Doppler ultrasonography – peripheral vascular disease.
e. Echocardiography – valvular heart disease.

94. In the posteroanterior chest radiograph, the heart shadow:

a. Will show left atrial enlargement.
b. Is increased in right ventricular hypertrophy.
c. Will show enlargement in hypertension.
d. Is normally about 50% of the transthoracic diameter.
e. Becomes enlarged in aortic stenosis.

95. Concerning cardiac enzymes:

a. An increase in creatine kinase always indicates a myocardial infarction.
b. Aspartate aminotransferase (AST) is also raised in liver disease.
c. Electrocardiographic testing is not required if cardiac enzymes are raised.
d. Lactate dehydrogenase reaches a peak within 24 hours.
e. Troponin T tests are not as specific as the tests for cardiac enzymes.

96. Electrocardiography:

a. Involves the use of ultrasound waves to map the heart.
b. Is not very good for looking at the movement of the heart and valves.
c. Cannot be used for the diagnosis of dilated cardiomyopathy.
d. Shows blood and fluid as a bright white colour.
e. Can use the Doppler shift to look at blood flow through valves.

97. Concerning the ECG and leads:

a. Lead aVL is a bipolar lead.
b. Conventionally the ECG is recorded using 12 leads.
c. Depolarization towards an electrode causes a positive deflection.
d. Lead aVF is placed on the axis at +90°.
e. The P wave represents atrial repolarization.

98. Concerning the ECG and rhythms:

a. Atrial fibrillation displays an absence of P waves.
b. In right bundle branch block, there is a Q wave with an S wave in V1.
c. In second degree heart block the QRS complexes are independent of P waves.
d. In ventricular fibrillation, the rhythm is irregular in amplitude but not rate.
e. In left bundle branch block there is a narrowing of the QRS complex.

99. Concerning the ECG and abnormalities:

a. Hyperkalaemia causes tall T waves and wide QRS complexes.
b. Hypocalcaemia causes a shortening of the QT interval.
c. S1Q3T3 is a feature of pulmonary embolism.
d. ST elevation in leads II, III and aVF represents an inferior myocardial infarction.
e. In right bundle branch block, there is a narrowing of the QRS complex.

100. Concerning the ECG and its recording:

a. The paper speed is usually 25 mm/s.
b. The RT interval can be used to calculate ventricular rate.
c. The normal PR interval is <100 ms.
d. Lead V_4 is usually over the interventricular septum.
e. The QT interval is approximately 500 ms.

Short-answer questions

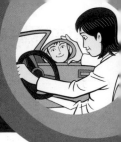

1. Outline the functions of the heart and cardiovascular system.

2. Outline the risk factors for ischaemic heart disease, and relate these to available treatments.

3. Describe the four most common congenital cardiac lesions.

4. Briefly describe the mechanism by which noradrenaline increases intracellular Ca^{2+} concentration in vascular smooth muscle cells.

5. Blood flows through a straight vessel of radius (r) 0.1 cm and length 1.0 cm at a rate of 0.03 mL/min. At the input end the pressure, P_a, is 90 mmHg and at the outflow end, P_v, is 10 mmHg.

   a. What will be the new flow if r increases to 0.2 cm with everything else constant?
   b. What will be the new flow if the viscosity of the blood increases by 50% with everything else held constant at the original values?
   c. What factors contribute to the viscosity of blood?
   d. What will be the new flow if P_a falls to 50 mmHg with everything else constant at the original values?

6.
   a. Explain what is meant by the term autoregulation.
   b. Give an example of a vascular bed that shows good autoregulation.
   c. What is the physiological importance of autoregulation in the tissue you have chosen?

7. Describe the carotid sinus baroreceptor reflex.

8.
   a. What is meant by the term vasoactive metabolite?
   b. Give two examples of vasoactive metabolites.
   c. Give an example of a situation in which they are important.

9.
   a. What is meant by the term stroke volume?
   b. Give the average value of end-diastolic volume of the left ventricle in a normal adult.
   c. Give the average value of end-systolic volume of the left ventricle in a normal adult.
   d. Give the average value of stroke volume of the left ventricle in a normal adult.
   e. What factors determine the stroke volume?
   f. What equations link: 1. Stroke volume to cardiac output; 2. Stroke volume to stroke work.

10.
   a. Explain how β-adrenoceptor antagonists (β-blockers) act on the cardiovascular system to relieve the symptoms of angina of effort.
   b. Why are β-blockers not used to treat vasospastic angina (Prinzmetal's angina)?

11.
   a. What is meant by the terms inotropic and chronotropic?
   b. Give an example of a positive chronotropic agent.

12. Outline how:
   a. Muscle blood flow is increased during exercise.
   b. Skin blood flow in the hand is reduced in cold weather.

13. Outline the factors that aid venous return from the feet during standing.

14. Describe the ECG changes which occur during a myocardial infarction.

15. List the signs and symptoms of heart failure, and the compensatory mechanisms which occur as a result.

16. Outline the role of the lymphatic system.

17. Describe the mechanism of the renin–angiotensin–aldosterone system.

18. Outline the factors influencing movement across the capillary endothelium.

19. Summarize the circulatory adaptations which occur at birth.

20. Outline the principles of:
   a. coronary artery bypass grafting (CABG).
   b. percutaneous transluminal coronary angioplasty (PTCA).

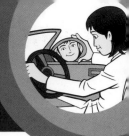

1. Match the following descriptions of chest pain to the correct diagnosis:

1. Myocardial infarction.
2. Oesophagitis.
3. Pulmonary embolism.
4. Angina.
5. Spontaneous pneumothorax.
6. Unstable angina.
7. Pericarditis.
8. Thoracic aortic dissection.
9. Oesophageal spasm.
10. Pneumonia.

A. A tall 22-year-old male on his way home from college suffered an episode of acute onset sharp chest pain which was worse on inspiration. ☐

B. A 57-year-old male lawyer who had smoked for 40 years complained of a sudden onset crushing central chest pain that radiated to his jaw. He felt sweaty and nauseous, and vomited on his way to the emergency department. ☐

C. A 29-year-old woman with systemic lupus erythematosus has been complaining of a few episodes of chest pain for the last week. The pain is worse on leaving forwards and on inspiration, but is relieved by ibuprofen. ☐

D. A 78-year-old retired postman complains of a sudden onset tearing central chest pain which radiates to his back between the shoulder blades. ☐

E. A 62-year-old factory worker with previous episodes of central chest pain brought on by walking his dog now complains of similar pain when he is sitting down reading the newspaper. ☐

2. Identify the most likely cause of shock from the scenarios below:

1. Anaphylaxis.
2. Sepsis.
3. Tension pneumothorax.
4. Haemorrhage.
5. Overdose.
6. Arrhythmia.
7. Myocardial infarction.
8. Pulmonary embolism.
9. Severe burns.
10. Dehydration.

A. A 62-year old-obese lady who is currently recovering from a recent knee replacement experiences an episode of acute onset chest pain and dyspnoea. Her observation chart shows a rising pulse rate and falling blood pressure. ☐

B. An 82-year-old man from a nursing home is brought into the emergency department as he is confused and been acting strangely. He has warm peripheries, a temperature of 38.2°C, and smells strongly of foul urine. ☐

C. A 64-year-old male complains of feeling unwell, nausea and has vomited. On further questioning, he admits to a 50-minute history of central chest pain radiating to his jaw. He is tachycardic, and his blood pressure has started to fall. ☐

D. A 27-year-old male is involved in a motor-vehicle accident. He is cool, pale and sweaty. His vital signs and examination are initially normal. Twenty minutes later his abdomen becomes very tense and tender. ☐

E. A 54-year-old male returns from theatre following a routine hernia repair. He becomes drowsy, flushed, sweaty and experiences some difficulty breathing. ☐

3. Identify the correct drug group from the descriptions of actions and side effects below:

1. β-Blockers.
2. Ca^{2+} channel blockers.
3. K^+ channel agonists.
4. ACE inhibitors.
5. Thiazide diuretics.
6. K^+ sparing diuretics.
7. Loop diuretics.
8. Non-steroidal anti-inflammatories.
9. Antibiotics.
10. Cardiac glycosides.

A. A first line anti-hypertensive which may cause hypokalaemia when given alone. It acts at the distal convoluted tubule. ☐

B. A low dose of a drug in this class has been shown to protect against cardiovascular events. It acts on the COX pathway. ☐

C. These drugs may cause bradycardia and cool peripheries, leading to a deterioration in peripheral vascular disease. ☐

D. This class of drug inhibits the conversion of angiotensin I to angiotensin II. ☐

E. This class of drug is useful in treating endocarditis, and should be given prior to any form of surgery in those at risk. ☐

4. Identify the arrhythmia from the ECG descriptions below:

1. Ventricular fibrillation.
2. Complete heart block.
3. Supraventricular tachycardia.
4. Ventricular tachycardia.
5. Atrial fibrillation.
6. Atrial flutter.
7. First degree heart block.
8. Right bundle branch block.
9. Left bundle branch block.
10. Torsade de pointes.

A. Rate 127, irregular, absent P waves, QRS duration 180 ms. ☐

B. Rate 150, regular, QRS duration 160 ms, saw-tooth appearance. ☐

C. Rate 90, regular, QRS duration 170 ms, PR interval 140 ms. ☐

D. Rate 180, regular, QRS duration 280 ms, monophasic pattern. ☐

E. Rate 100, regular, QRS duration 160 ms, PR interval 100 ms, P waves unrelated to QRS complexes. ☐

5. Match the following collection of signs and symptoms to the correct diagnosis:

1. Pulmonary embolism.
2. Myocardial infarction.
3. Heart failure.
4. Peripheral vascular disease.
5. Lymphoedema.
6. Lymphoma.
7. Varicose veins.
8. Pulmonary oedema.
9. Deep vein thrombosis.
10. Lymphangitis.

A. A 68-year-old gentleman with a history of ischaemic heart disease complains of dyspnoea, predominantly on exercise and when lying flat. He has also noticed some swelling of his calves. ☐

B. A 49-year-old diabetic complains of pain in his calves which comes on when walking and is relieved by rest. ☐

C. An 80-year-old lady complains of diffuse non-pitting oedema in both legs to the level of the thigh following pelvic surgery. ☐

D. A 64-year-old retired teacher who suffers from breast cancer complains of some unsightly swellings on her calves which occasionally bleed when knocked. ☐

E. A 47-year-old gentleman has recently returned from abroad and within hours is complaining of an aching, swelling and redness in his left calf. He was previously fit and well. ☐

6. Identify from the descriptions below the correct congenital defect:

1. Ventricular septal defect.
2. Transposition of the great arteries.
3. Coarctation of the aorta.
4. Atrial septal defect.
5. Patent ductus arteriosus.
6. Eisenmenger's syndrome.
7. Berry aneurysm.
8. Aortic aneurysm.
9. Tetralogy of Fallot.
10. Atrioventricular septal defect.

A. This is caused by a failure of closure of the foramen ovale. There is a fixed, widely split second heart sound on auscultation. ☐

B. This is identified by an ejection systolic murmur, usually heard best on the back, and weak femoral pulses. ☐

C. This is a cyanotic heart lesion which develops later on in life. ☐

D. This lesion is pathognomonic of Down syndrome. ☐

E. Infundibular pulmonary stenosis is one component of this lesion. ☐

7. Match the following signs to the correct diagnosis:

1. Atrial myxoma.
2. Aortic stenosis.
3. Turner's syndrome.
4. Mitral stenosis.
5. Marfan syndrome.
6. Hyperlipidaemia.
7. Aortic regurgitation.
8. Infective endocarditis.
9. Diabetes.
10. Hypertension.

A. Osler's nodes. ☐
B. Malar flush. ☐
C. High arched palate. ☐
D. Collapsing pulse. ☐
E. Corneal arcus. ☐

8. Match the following description of skin lesions to the correct diagnosis:

1. Venous ulcer.
2. Basal cell carcinoma.
3. Arterial ulcer.
4. Marjolin's ulcer.
5. Squamous cell carcinoma.
6. Gangrene.
7. Neuropathic ulcer.
8. Traumatic ulcer.
9. Diabetic ulcer.
10. Malignant melanoma.

A. A shallow, sloughy ulcer on the medial malleolus of the calf. ☐
B. A 4 mm well circumscribed ulcer between the toes. The limb has no foot pulses below the femoral artery. Sensation remains intact. ☐
C. A 5 mm ulcer with a raised, pearly edge. ☐
D. A 7 mm lesion on the sole of a 54 year old diabetic male. The food has good pulses, and sensation remains intact. ☐
E. A 3 mm ulcer on the heel, noticed initially on removal of a plaster cast. The cast was placed several weeks earlier for an ankle fracture. ☐

9. Select the most appropriate definitive investigation for the conditions listed below:

1. D dimer.
2. Venography.
3. Echocardiogram.
4. Chest x-ray.
5. Arterial duplex.
6. CT scan.
7. CT-pulmonary angiogram.
8. Troponin I (at 2 hours).
9. ECG.
10. Ventilation/perfusion (VQ) scan.

A. Pulmonary embolism. ☐
B. Myocardial infarction. ☐
C. Deep vein thrombosis. ☐
D. Congestive cardiac failure. ☐
E. Peripheral vascular disease. ☐

10. Match the following descriptions to the correct cardiac murmur:

1. Mitral stenosis.
2. Austin Flint murmur.
3. Pulmonary stenosis.
4. Ventricular septal defect.
5. Aortic stenosis.
6. Patent ductus arteriosus.
7. Aortic regurgitation.
8. Mitral regurgitation.
9. Tricuspid regurgitation.
10. Graham Steele murmur.

A. A high pitched, pansystolic murmur heard loudest at the apex. ☐
B. A continuous systolic and diastolic murmur heard best just below the clavicle. ☐
C. A harsh ejection systolic murmur which radiates to the carotids. ☐
D. A low pitched rumbling diastolic murmur heard only with the bell. ☐
E. A quiet, end-diastolic murmur heard best in expiration at the lower left sternal edge. The patient has a widened pulse pressure. ☐

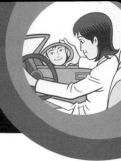

1.
a. True   The cardiovascular system is responsible for transporting metabolites in plasma, including glucose and lipids.
b. True   Many hormones are soluble factors carried in the blood.
c. True   Local regulation of blood flow plays a key role in inflammation; immune cells and cytokines are carried in blood and lymph.
d. True   Temperature regulation is achieved by regulation of the circulation of the skin.
e. True   The cardiovascular system is responsible for an erection.

2.
a. False   The pulmonary vein is one of two exceptions to the rule and this carries oxygenated blood to the heart.
b. True   The heart is responsible for the secretion of hormones, e.g. atrial natriuretic peptide.
c. False   The pulmonary vasculature has a lower resistance resulting in lower pressures.
d. True   The pressure diminishes the further away from the heart the vessel runs.
e. True   Although this can vary; if it becomes inadequate, renal failure may result.

3.
a. True   The thymus lies anteriorly in the superior and inferior mediastinum.
b. False   It is the base of the pericardium which fuses with the diaphragm.
c. True   Although the right ventricle lies anteriorly.
d. True   This is a very important clinical landmark.
e. True   Two – returning blood from each lung merge to form the left atrium.

4.
a. False   The mitral valve has two cusps (bicuspid), although this location is correct.
b. False   There is one left and one right, although the left coronary artery bifurcates early.
c. True   This is distinct from the atrioventricular valves.
d. True   They are some of the earliest branches.
e. False   The coronary veins drains into the coronary sinus and then into the right atrium.

5.
a. False   Development of the heart begins in week 3 of gestation.
b. False   The septum spurium is purely transient, while the septum primum and septum secundum separate the atria.
c. True   The truncus arteriosus undergoes a spiral process of septation to split the aorta and pulmonary trunk before rotating and separating.
d. True   The superior part of the interventricular septum is a membranous extension of the fibrous skeleton of the heart.
e. True   The single pulmonary vein becomes four through intussusception incorporating the first two branch points into the atrial wall.

6.
a. True   This is important as it makes them at risk of endocarditis.
b. True   These muscles ensure competency of the valves, preventing regurgitation.
c. True   As the valves are avascular, this is the only possible route; diffusion.
d. False   Rheumatic fever most commonly targets the mitral valve.
e. True   This is one of the four features of this condition.

7.
a. True   The resting membrane potential of contractile myocytes is –90 mV, predominantly through the concentration gradient of K^+ ions.
b. False   The developed tension in myocytes is proportional to cytoplasmic Ca^{2+} concentration, and so positive inotropes raise Ca^{2+} levels.
c. False   Intercalated disks form the structural junctions between myocytes while the gap junctions allow rapid electrical conduction.
d. True   Nodal, Purkinje fibre and work cells are all examples of specialized myocytes.
e. True   The membrane potential of pacemaker cells declines partly through the leakage of Na^+ ions to threshold, when Ca^{2+} channels open.

8.
a. True   The resting membrane potential is maintained through the K^+ gradient, with Na^+ movement initiating depolarization.

b. True   Contractile myocytes are most permeable to K^+ ions.

c. False   The upstroke in nodal cells is relatively slow, and is dependent on an influx of Ca^{2+} ions.

d. False   The Nernst equation predicts the membrane potential resulting from an ionic concentration gradient.

e. False   In work myocytes, the upstroke is mediated by movement of Na^+ ions.

9. a. True   Raised cytosolic Ca^{2+} triggers contraction.

b. True   An increased heart rate reduces the time for removal of cytoplasmic Ca^{2+} leading to raised levels of Ca^{2+} and, therefore, increased force.

c. True   Tension, or force of contraction, is proportional to cytoplasmic Ca^{2+} levels.

d. True   Changes that produce a higher resting Ca^{2+} level will lead to an increased force of contraction.

e. False   Chronotropes affect the heart rate, not the strength of contraction.

10. a. True   This is initially passive and then active.

b. True   The coronary arteries fill as the ventricles relax during diastole.

c. False   The presence of atrial systole and contraction is not essential, although ventricular filling is reduced in atrial fibrillation.

d. True   It is caused by the closing of atrioventricular valves.

e. True   As ventricular pressure falls during diastole the valve opens.

11. a. False   The force of contraction is directly proportional to the initial length of the muscle fibre.

b. False   Starling's law was first described in studies on isolated heart–lung preparations but is also valid physiologically.

c. True   The EDV determines the initial fibre length. This determines the force of contraction and hence the stroke volume.

d. False   Factors that reduce cardiac filling will reduce EDV and hence reduce the force of contraction.

e. False   Starling's law reflects the intrinsic properties of cardiac myocytes, and does not depend on innervation.

12. a. False   Cardiac output is the product of stroke volume and heart rate.

b. True   Contractility is affected by factors such as sympathetic stimulation.

c. True   End-diastolic volume and end-diastolic pressure are closely related because the relaxed ventricle stretches in response to increased pressure.

d. False   The Starling curve has a peak, but the downslope is caused by architectural distortion of the heart. Individual myocytes cannot be overstretched, unlike skeletal muscle.

e. True   This relation is the physiological equivalent of Ohm's law (i.e. resistance = pressure divided by flow).

13. a. False   This is ventricular repolarization; atrial repolarization is masked in the QRS complex.

b. True   This can be calculated easily from the ECG rhythm strip.

c. True   The peak of the R wave coincides with depolarization of the apex.

d. True   A PR interval of 120–200 ms is normal.

e. False S_1 occurs with ventricular contraction, i.e. just after the QRS complex.

14. a. True   This reflects the change in function of these vessels.

b. True   This is the main source of return of blood to the heart.

c. False   The large vessels also receive nutrients via the vasa vasorum in the adventitia.

d. True   There are, however, exchange vessels in addition to these in the portal circulation.

e. False   It is larger than this, approximately 25 mm.

15. a. False   The brachial artery is a continuation of the axillary artery.

b. True   This contributes to the elastic nature of the vessel.

c. True   These vessels supply the head, neck and upper limbs.

d. False   The coronary arteries come off the aorta just above the aortic valve.

e. True   This is important in understanding the anatomy of abdominal aortic aneurysms.

16. a. False   The coeliac trunk supplies the foregut structures; mid-gut structures are supplied by the superior mesenteric artery.

b. False   This is a branch of the hepatic artery.

c. True   These are multiple arteries which branch off the inferior mesenteric artery.

d. True   These are mid-gut structures.

e. True   The left gastric artery supplies the lesser curvature of the stomach.

17. a. False   The complete circle ensure limited neurological deficit in stroke patients.

b. True   This is commonly affected in cerebrovascular disease.

c. True   The external jugular vein joins the internal jugular vein on its return to the heart.

d. False   The facial artery is a branch of the external carotid artery.

e. True   The tributaries drain to the superior vena cava and then the right atrium.

18. a. True   As the lungs fill with air, pulmonary resistance falls rapidly to allow greater volumes of blood to flow.

b. False   During fetal development atrial pressures are equal, but the left atria develops a higher pressure after birth.

c. True   Prostaglandins maintain the patency of the ductus venosus during gestation.

d. False   There is no real rush to clamp the cord, although it should be done correctly as the neonate may exsanguinate through an incompletely clamped cord.

e. True   The increased left atrial pressure seals the septum primum over the foramen ovale.

19. a. True   The intracellular binding site for EDRF is on guanyl cyclase.

b. True   Adrenaline binds to cell surface receptors, which activate adenylase cyclase.

c. True   The transmitter used in sympathetic neuromuscular junctions is noradrenaline.

d. True   Hypoxia causes hyperpolarization which reduces the number of open Ca^{2+} channels and hence reduces contraction.

e. False   Smooth muscle is able to maintain tension for only 0.3% of the energy requirement of skeletal muscle.

20. a. True   The higher the stroke volume, the greater the pressure wave.

b. True   The lower the heart rate, the greater the pressure wave.

c. True   The more elastic the artery, the greater the pressure wave.

d. True   The higher the peripheral resistance, the greater the pressure wave.

e. True   The higher the blood volume, the greater the pressure wave.

21. a. True   This is due to lack of elasticity which develops in the vessels.

b. False   Blood pressure is measured in mmHg.

c. True   The mean gives a better marker of beat-to-beat organ perfusion.

d. False   Blood pressure falls because of the body's decreased metabolic demands.

e. True   Occasionally IV is used, for example, in pregnancy.

22. a. True   Flow varies with the pressure difference and the resistance.

b. False   Poiseuille's law determines resistance, such that flow is proportional to the radius to the fourth power.

c. False   Similarly, flow is inversely proportional to the length (resistance is proportional to length).

d. True   Increasing the velocity increases the resistance and hence decreases flow.

e. True   Flow is defined as the volume of blood flowing per unit time, and is, therefore, dependent on velocity.

23. a. False   This is a dynamic process, with continuing cycling of clot.

b. True   Although it may be initiated by platelet aggregation or plasma protein activation.

c. True   Haemophilia A is a bleeding diasthesis which is hereditary and X-linked.

d. False   It is common but results in a hypercoagulable state.

e. True   Thrombocythaemia is a strong risk factor for thrombosis.

24. a. False   Central venous pressure is lower than in the periphery, at around 0–6 mmHg.

b. True   This is results in venoconstriction and maintenance of tone.

c. False   Orthostasis causes an increased blood pressure in any vessel below the heart.

d. True   The increase in venous return on skeletal muscle contraction causes a rise in central venous pressure.

e. False   Flow increases due to a fall in intrathoracic pressure.

25. a. False   Veins contain about 60% of total blood volume. The capillaries only hold the blood involved in direct exchange.

b. True   Red blood cells are forced to deform as they pass through the smallest capillaries to maximize gaseous exchange.

c. True   Capillary sphincters control capillary blood flow, but do not contribute to resistance.

d. True   Capillary walls also allow diffusion of water soluble molecules.

e. False   Capillary walls are incapable of vasoconstriction. The arterioles are the resistance vessels.

26. a. True   This ensures adequate fluid exchange. The converse is true at the venous end of the capillary.

b. True   It is 37 mmHg at the arterial end and 17 mmHg at the venous end.

c. True   This is the basis of Love's simplification of Laplace's law.

d. False   This occurs by diffusion.

e. False   Hypoproteinaemia results in an decrease in osmotic pressure and subsequent oedema.

27. a. True   Extracellular or interstitial fluid is drained via the lymphatics.

b. False   Lymph returns to the circulation through the subclavian vein.

c. True   Lymphatic drainage ensures that antigens from the interstitial fluid are screened in lymph nodes.

d. False   Lymph carries fats absorbed from the gut to the central circulation.

e. False   Both brain and eye are unique in having their own systems for drainage.

28. a. False   Hyperpolarization mediates smooth muscle relaxation in response to hypoxia.

b. True   Autoregulation is the process whereby vessel calibre automatically adapts to changes in perfusion pressure.

c. False   Hyperaemia may be pathological, but is also physiological, e.g. in exercising muscle.

d. False   There are sympathetic afferents which mediate vasodilatation in skeletal muscle.

e. True   There are no parasympathetic vasoconstrictor nerves.

29. a. False   Renin is released from the juxtaglomerular cells in the kidney.

b. True   First discovered in extracts of brain tissue, brain natriuretic peptide is released from the ventricles in response to stretch.

c. True   Vasopressin, otherwise known as anti-diuretic hormone (ADH), is released in response to an increased osmolarity.

d. False   Angiotensin I is converted to angiotensin II by endothelial cells in the lung. Angiotensin II leads to vasoconstriction.

e. True   Aldosterone acts on the renal tubules of the kidney to promote Na^+ and water retention.

30. a. True   It may be rest by autonomic activity in, e.g. exercise, and also responds to flow and metabolic demand.

b. True   increased pressures leads to greater tension in the vessel wall in order to increase resistance and regulate flow.

c. False   Autoregulation acts to maintain constant flow at varying pressure, but is sensitive to metabolic demand.

d. False   Myogenic autoregulation is achieved by the smooth muscle of the arterial walls and does not rely on innervation.

e. False   The hyperpolarization and smooth muscle relaxation induced by hypoxia is a form of autoregulation.

31. a. False   The responses to a fall in blood pressure act to maintain the blood flow to critical organs (e.g. the brain), by vasodilatation.

b. True   Vessels supplying skeletal muscle and other peripheral organs will vasoconstrict.

c. True   Venoconstriction occurs by sympathetic activation to increase venous return and maintain cardiac output.

d. False   Chemoreceptors in the aortic and carotid bodies will respond to a reduced blood pressure by stimulating ventilation.

e. True   The baroreceptor response to reduced blood pressure includes increased sympathetic activation which increases cardiac contractility.

32. a. True   Despite being so important, it receives only a relatively small amount.

b. False   The metabolic demand of the brain changes very little.

c. True   This prolongs aerobic respiration in the muscles.

d. False   The high flow is a result of the kidneys specialized role in excretion.

e. False   The kidneys have the highest blood flow per 100 g.

33. a. False   Adrenaline is secreted from the adrenal medulla.

b. False   Renin is the enzyme which catalyses the conversion of angiotensinogen to angiotensin I.

c. False   ACE is predominantly found in the vasculature of the lung.

d. True   This results in increased water retention by the kidney.

e. True   This is due to the presence and high affinity for β-receptors.

34. a. True   This is as a result of vasodilatation and an increased pressure gradient.

b. True   This occurs as a result of increased heart rate, cardiac filling and contractility.

c. False   This would occur in heart failure; in exercise the cavity is increased but the wall is thick.

d. True   Peripheral vessels initially contract to maintain blood pressure, but dilate as core temperature rises.

e. False   The exercise pressor response stimulates cardiac output in response to exercise, not the Starling mechanism.

35. a. False   Disorders causing pro-coagulative states, however, are a risk factor.

b. True   This is a strong risk factor.

c. True   This implies decreased oestrogen exposure, which is protective from ischaemic heart disease.

d. True   Although this is likely to be a confounding factor.

e. True   Excess platelet production leads to increased blood viscosity.

36. a. True   This permits more time spent in diastole and better myocardial perfusion.

b. True   The implication of this is that is should be used cautiously with β-blockers.

c. False   Drugs ending in '-pril' belong to the group of ACE inhibitors.

d. False   These side effects are classic of β-blockers.

e. True   This is because it is rapidly absorbed from here and subject to first-pass metabolism.

37. a. False   The left anterior descending artery (a branch of the left coronary artery) is usually responsible.

b. False   This may occur, but as a late complication.

c. False   Irreversible damage occurs after 20–40 minutes.

d. True   This is variable however, and follows the granulation stage.

e. True   Acute events are usually initiated by acute changes in plaques.

38. a. True   Usually as a result of ventricular fibrillation.

b. False   The mitral valve is usually affected secondary to papillary muscle infarction.

c. True   Cerebrovascular accident and recurrent myocardial infarction are frequent sequelae of acute MI.

d. False   These pathologies are unrelated.

e. True   This may be a mural thrombus although MI patients are also more prone to deep vein thrombosis (DVT).

39. a. True   This affects the Starling curve in heart failure, decreasing cardiac output.

b. False   Excretion of K^+ occurs; it is Na^+ and water which are retained leading to oedema.

c. True   These findings are typical of a failing chamber.

d. False   Shortness of breath is more pronounced when lying flat, known as orthopnoea.

e. True   They should be in all patients, but care taking when co-prescribing diuretics.

40. a. True   It is a frequent cause in the young.

b. True   Although this has a minimal effect on cardiac output.

c. False   The pulse in atrial fibrillation is irregular in both rate and volume.

d. True   This is the diagnostic criteria, an absence of coordinated atrial activity.

e. True   This is the most effective in new-onset atrial fibrillation.

41. a. False   This is a non-specific finding, and may arise from supraventricular or ventricular tachycardia.

b. False   Carotid sinus massage may slow a tachycardia but does not differentiate supraventricular from ventricular causes.

c. True   There is a degree of atrioventricular dissociation, resulting in this abnormality of the jugular venous waveform.

d. True   Ventricular tachycardia is usually found in the presence of cardiac failure.

e. True   This is a non-specific finding with tachycardia, but does indicate a ventricular origin.

42. a. False   Supraventricular arrhythmias may originate from anywhere 'above the ventricle', not confined to the atrioventricular node.

b. False   Heart rates are considered normal between 60 and 100 beats per minute, although athletes may have a lower resting pulse.

c. True   Sinus arrhythmia, a change in heart rate with respiration, is normal in the young.

d. True   Wolf–Parkinson–White syndrome is caused by an extra conduction pathway and frequently causes tachycardia or atrial fibrillation.

e. True   There is delayed conduction between the atria and the ventricles leading to an increased PR interval.

43. a. True   Amiodarone may cause a fibrosing alveolitis.

b. True   Many drugs may cause liver damage in individual patients.

c. False   Constipation is a side effect of verapamil.

d. False   Exacerbation of asthma is a risk accompanying the use of β-blockers.

e. True   Amiodarone contains iodine and is a recognized cause of thyroid disorders.

44. a. True   Overexertion of the heart beyond the available blood supply creates ischaemia.

b. False   Unstable angina is a serious condition, as 15% of cases progress to a myocardial infarction. Classical angina of effort is not life-threatening.

c. True   Atheromatous changes are the most common cause of stenosis.

d. False   Treatment for angina aims to reduce the work of the heart and increase the coronary blood flow.

e. True   Verapamil blocks Ca^{2+} channels, producing vasodilatation and reducing arterial resistance.

45. a. False   ST elevation may occur within the first few hours of myocardial infarction, if it is going to appear at all.

b. True   The affected region of the heart may rupture up to several days after a myocardial infarction causing cardiac tamponade.

c. True   Platelet aggregation or thrombosis from an atherosclerotic lesion are frequent causes of myocardial infarction.

d. True   Incomplete vessel occlusion may produce a sub-endocardial infarct that progresses with complete occlusion.

e. True   Reperfusion injury occurs when blood flow is re-established, and so there may be further loss of myocytes after thrombolysis.

46. a. False   A normal pericardium may contain 50 mL of fluid.

b. True   Effusions may arise from blood, interstitial fluid or lymph.

c. True   Cardiac tamponade prevents adequate cardiac filling and must be drained.

d. True   Pericarditis occurs in 30% of patients with severe, chronic rheumatoid arthritis.

e. False   Serous effusions result from heart failure or hypoproteinaemia, whilst infected effusions are usually purulent.

47. a. True   Cough is a recognized respiratory cause of syncope.

b. True   A tumour that exerts pressure on or invades the aorta may produce syncope.

c. True   Syncope associated with arrhythmia (Stokes-Adams attacks) are associated with pallor, followed by facial flushing as the cardiac output is restored.

d. True   The most common cause of fainting is a vasovagal attack, triggered by pain or other emotional stimulus.

e. False   Mitral regurgitation is not associated with syncope on exertion.

48. a. False   The term cardiomyopathy is generally used for conditions where the pathogenesis is unknown.

b. True   Cardiomyopathy is classified in this way.

c. False   Restrictive cardiomyopathy is associated with stiffening of a normal size ventricular wall.

d. True   Chronic, excessive levels of catecholamines may lead to dilated cardiomyopathy.

e. True   Excessive dilatation leads to poor cardiac function, which may lead to heart failure, mural thrombi, or arrhythmias.

49. a. True   Current schemes classify the disease according to the infective organism.

b. True   Oral or pharyngeal pathogens may enter the bloodstream after dental treatment.

c. True   Intravenous drug users risk introducing pathogenic organisms into their blood.

d. True   Non-bacterial thrombotic endocarditis may arise through clotting disorders.

e. True   Sequelae of endocarditis include valve incompetence, embolic disease and renal complications.

50. a. True   Streptococcal septicaemia is a common precursor to rheumatic fever.

b. True   Erythema marginatum (a macular rash with an erythematous edge) occurs more frequently in children.

c. True   Rheumatic fever is an autoimmune, systemic inflammatory disease. The ESR is frequently raised.

d. False   The joint pain in rheumatic fever typically affects the large joints.

e. False   Rheumatic fever is associated with small, bead-like vegetations on heart valves.

51. a. True   This is correct. Some symptomatic improvement in the severity of the angina is also usually gained.
    b. True   Re-stenosis may occur after both angioplasty and CABG, but at a lower incidence following CABG.
    c. False Grafts are taken from the patient's own vasculature.
    d. False Bypass grafting is usually only offered to patients with severe or refractory angina.
    e. True   Both CABG and angioplasty result in a reduction in the need for anti-anginals.

52. a. True   Primary cardiac tumours are extremely rare.
    b. True   Myxomatous masses may fragment to produce emboli.
    c. False 75% of cardiac myxomas arise in the left atrium.
    d. True   Echocardiography is a useful and non-invasive investigation to visualize the heart.
    e. True   Systemic responses to cancer may lead to non-bacterial thrombotic endocarditis.

53. a. False Ventricular septal defects account for approximately 30% of all congenital heart lesions.
    b. True   Only 10% will require drug therapy or surgery.
    c. True   This is because there is flow across the duct in both systole and diastole.
    d. False The shunt is left ventricle to right ventricle, therefore the murmur is systolic.
    e. True   Although it is still less common than VSD in these children.

54. a. True   Usually distal to the subclavian artery resulting in upper limb hypertension.
    b. True   Although this is not present in all cases, there is a strong association.
    c. False Weak femoral pulses are present with strong radial pulses.
    d. False This is much rarer, the figure is nearer 7%.
    e. False These symptoms are classic of aortic stenosis.

55. a. True   This is incompatible with life in the absence of another lesion allowing mixing of systemic and pulmonary blood.

b. False   This occurs from pulmonary hypertension caused by increased pulmonary blood flow.
c. False   The only treatment for Eisenmenger's syndrome is heart–lung transplantation.
d. False   Right ventricular hypertrophy occurs as a result of pulmonary stenosis.
e. True   Cyanotic heart disease is one of the cardiac causes of clubbing.

56. a. False This occurs from myocardial or aortic rupture.
    b. False 200–300 mL fluid is sufficient to cause cardiac tamponade.
    c. True   These commonly leave adhesions when healed.
    d. True   Pancarditis is a major feature of rheumatic fever.
    e. True   This refers to an increase in jugular venous pressure on inspiration.

57. a. True   Any of these organisms may cause myocarditis.
    b. False Dilatation occurs in all four chambers.
    c. True   Both central and peripheral thrombosis.
    d. True   Dyspnoea, chest pain and arrhythmias may all be features of myocarditis.
    e. False Treatment of myocarditis should be directed at the underlying cause.

58. a. False Shock can result from haemorrhage, dehydration, anaphylaxis and many other causes.
    b. True   The body compensates for fluid loss by retention of water and Na^+.
    c. False Cardiogenic shock from chronic heart failure should not be treated with adrenaline.
    d. True   Physiological compensatory mechanisms initially defend blood pressure.
    e. True   Sympathetic activation to maintain cardiac output and blood pressure results in peripheral vasoconstriction.

59. a. True   Platelet derived growth factor (PDGF) released by adherent platelets is a smooth muscle mitogen.
    b. True   Smooth muscle cell migration from the media into the intima is a key pathogenic step.
    c. True   Macrophages are recruited into the atherosclerotic lesion where they oxidize LDL and secrete growth factors.
    d. True   Atherosclerotic changes are likely to be initiated by endothelial injury.
    e. True   Many cytokines are involved in the recruitment and multiplication of cells in atherosclerotic lesions.

60.
a. False   α-Adrenoreceptors mediate constriction in the vasculature, and so should be blocked.

b. True   Methyldopa is a centrally acting antihypertensive reserved for use in pregnancy.

c. True   Cyanide poisoning is a risk with long-term use of sodium nitroprusside in patients with renal failure, although this is rarely a practical problem.

d. True   Potassium channel agonists hyperpolarize smooth muscle cells, producing vasodilatation.

e. False   Angiotensin II receptor antagonists can be tried if ACE inhibitors produce an intolerable cough by elevating levels of bradykinin.

61.
a. True   Lipoproteins are composed of lipids and apolipoproteins. The apolipoproteins have several roles.

b. True   Oxidized LDL is likely to play a significant role in attracting macrophages into the atherosclerotic lesions.

c. True   Type I hyperlipidaemia is characterized by raised triglyceride levels alone, and is treated by dietary control.

d. False   Statins inhibit HMG CoA reductase, which is involved in endogenous synthesis of cholesterol. They have no effect on triglyceride levels.

e. False   Fibrates act on adipose tissue to reduce activity of lipoprotein lipase.

62.
a. True   Urine output is minimized to reduce fluid loss.

b. True   Sympathetic activation leads to sweating and peripheral vasoconstriction.

c. True   Increased thirst is part of the physiological response to fluid loss.

d. True   Total peripheral resistance is increased to maintain blood pressure and maintain essential organ perfusion.

e. False   Tachycardia is a common sign in haemorrhagic shock.

63.
a. True   Raised cholesterol is a major feature of type II hypercholesterolaemia.

b. False   High levels of HDL are protective against atherosclerosis and coronary heart disease.

c. False   High levels of triglycerides may lead to pancreatitis.

d. True   Diabetes mellitus has many effects on metabolism.

e. False   Statins act on HMG CoA reductase to reduce endogenous cholesterol synthesis.

64.
a. False   The definition of hypertension also depends on age; higher limits are set for blood pressure in the elderly.

b. False   Causes of hypertension are diverse and multifactorial.

c. True   ACE inhibitors are widely used in the treatment of hypertension.

d. False   Reduction of blood pressure, even within the range defined as normal, will reduce mortality.

e. True   Normal physiological defence of blood pressure weakens with age.

65.
a. True   Extension of the tear towards the valves may disrupt their function.

b. True   Chest pain with radiation to the back suggests aortic dissection.

c. False   Surgery is the definitive treatment for a dissecting aortic aneurysm, but there may or may not be a re-entry point.

d. True   Computerized tomography using contrast medium is the optimal imaging technique.

e. True   Aortic aneurysms are a recognised complication of syphilis.

66.
a. True   Giant cell (temporal) arteritis may also lead to blindness.

b. True   20% of patients will have coronary arteritis with aneurysms.

c. False   Polyarteritis nodosa more commonly affects the small to medium size arteries.

d. True   Necrotizing vasculitis of the lungs and glomerulonephritis forms part of the classical presentation.

e. False   Thromboangiitis obliterans usually affects young men who smoke.

67.
a. True   Haemangiomas are common, especially in children.

b. True   Ulcerated haemangiomas are known as granuloma pyogenicum and affect 5% of pregnant women.

c. True   Juvenile capillary haemangiomas appear at birth, but usually disappear by age 5 years.

d. False   Capillary haemangiomas may also occur in mucosal membranes.

e. True   Haemangiomas make up approximately 7% of all benign tumours.

68.
a. True   Many patients with DVT have ankle oedema because of reduced venous outflow from the leg.

b. True   Fever is a recognized sign of pulmonary embolism.

c. True   Doppler ultrasonography is useful to identify blocked vessels.

d. True   Primary or secondary pulmonary tumours may give rise to the symptoms of pulmonary embolism.

e. False   Lifelong treatment may be indicated in certain circumstances, e.g. hypercoagulable states or repeated episodes.

69.
a. True   Although this occurs as a late sign.

b. True   Although this occurs as a late sign.

c. False   A narrowing of the pulse pressure is seen as the diastolic pressure rises.

d. False   Urine output falls as a result of underperfusion of the kidneys.

e. True   This may occur, particularly in sepsis and anaphylaxis.

70.
a. True   This is predominantly a direct result of vasoconstriction.

b. False   This does occur, but as a late response.

c. True   This stimulates an increase in angiotensin II and aldosterone.

d. True   This is the starting point for the cascade of events which follow.

e. True   This is one of a number of mechanisms promoting haemostasis of fluid balance.

71.
a. False   Abdominal aortic aneurysms are usually fusiform.

b. True   Although unfortunately the majority of these men are asymptomatic.

c. True   Hypertension is thought to be one of the biggest risk factors for both development and progression.

d. False   It is much closer to 50%.

e. False   They are usually infra-renal but above the iliac bifurcation.

72.
a. False   They are, by definition, permanent dilatations.

b. False   They may occur in the heart and even in the veins.

c. False   Although they may be caused by syphilis.

d. True   This is by far the most common aneurysm.

e. False   It is an aneurysm which occurs as the result of a tear in the arterial wall.

73.
a. True   This should be specifically sought on clinical examination of patients with chest pain.

b. False   The tear occurs in the media.

c. True   Type B arise from the arch and descending aorta.

d. False   There is no mortality benefit associated with surgery in these cases. Treatment is medical with lowering of blood pressure.

e. True   Blood may back track along the aorta leading to haemopericardium.

74.
a. False   This is a congenital abnormality of the atrial septum in the heart.

b. True   This is an uncommon abnormality and may also lead to compression of the trachea.

c. False   Hypoplasia of the lymphatic system is primary lymphoedema.

d. True   This may be congenital, or constructed surgically for the purposes of dialysis.

e. True   This would maintain renal perfusion in hypovolaemia.

75.
a. False   They are usually asymptomatic and only cause headache when they rupture.

b. False   They bleed into the subarachnoid space.

c. False   Rupture is more common in men aged 40–60.

d. False   They are caused by focal wall weakness which may occur anywhere in the circle of Willis.

e. True   Along with hypertension and atheroma.

76.
a. False   They are dilated, tortuous superficial veins.

b. False   These are risk factors for deep vein thrombosis.

c. True   This is a strong risk factor.

d. False   They should only be treated if symptomatic.

e. False   The walls become thin and distended.

77.
a. True   This creates a procoagulant state and leads to immobility.

b. True   Although calf swelling and tenderness is common.

c. True   This is literally migrating thrombi.

d. False   Warfarin may be used long term but initial treatment is with heparin.

e. False   It is highly unlikely that below-knee DVTs are more common than above-knee DVTS. Above-knee DVTs rarely cause symptoms however, and are therefore not normally identified.

78.
a. False   The pain is cramping in nature and relieved by rest.

b. True   This helps prevent thrombus formation and worsening of symptoms.

c. False   Smoking is a very strong risk factor.

d. False   These cause peripheral vasoconstriction and may exacerbate symptoms.

e. True   The same risk factors apply and the patient group is often the same.

79.
a. True — This predisposes to calf symptoms but may be easily treated.

b. False — Approximately 15% of the normal adult population have an absent foot pulse.

c. True — Arterial ulcers are painful, well demarcated and on the lateral aspect of the foot.

d. True — Diabetes is a strong risk factor for peripheral vascular disease.

e. False — Statins are useful to alter the lipid profile and prevent disease progression.

80.
a. True — Syncope may result from inadequate cerebral perfusion.

b. True — Visual impairment may also result from limited cerebral perfusion.

c. True — Nausea and vomiting may indicate malignant hypertension.

d. True — Paroxysmal nocturnal dyspnoea is an indication of right heart failure.

e. True — Neurological deficits may indicate a stroke or transient ischaemic attack.

81.
a. True — The pain of a dissecting aortic aneurysm is usually sharp and radiates towards the back.

b. True — Pulmonary emboli typically give rise to a localized, sharp chest pain.

c. True — The pain associated with a pneumothorax is usually felt laterally but may also cause central chest pain.

d. True — Oesophagitis commonly gives rise to a burning retrosternal pain.

e. True — The pain of pericarditis is usually associated with breathing or movement.

82.
a. True — This and ventricular tachycardia are both treatable with defibrillation.

b. True — This increases the effectiveness of resuscitation.

c. False — This should be reserved for patients with asystolic arrest or pulseless electrical activity with a rate <60 bpm.

d. True — Needle decompression would reduce intra-thoracic pressure and allow blood to return to the heart.

e. True — The patient would be neither breathing, nor have a pulse.

83.
a. True — Alternating strong and weak pulses indicate severe left ventricular disease.

b. True — Aortic constriction reduced maximum flow through the aortic valve.

c. False — A collapsing pulse is characteristic of aortic regurgitation.

d. True — A pulse that weakens or disappears on inspiration may be caused by asthma, pericarditis or tamponade.

e. False — A combination of slow rising and collapsing pulse indicates both aortic stenosis and regurgitation.

84.
a. True — The 'a' wave is caused by atrial contraction. Without coordinated activity this pressure wave does not occur.

b. False — Giant 'a' waves are an indication of tricuspid stenosis, not regurgitation.

c. False — Large 'v' waves are characteristic of tricuspid regurgitation, or constrictive pericarditis.

d. True — The 'y' descent corresponds with the opening of the tricuspid valve and is slow with a stenosed valve.

e. True — JVP is raised on inspiration with cardiac tamponade and constrictive pericarditis.

85.
a. False — The first heart sound occurs before ejection, and so will be heard before the pressure wave is palpable in the carotid artery.

b. False — Physiological splitting of the second heart sound is observed on inspiration.

c. True — The mid-diastolic click indicates the opening of an abnormal mitral or tricuspid valve.

d. True — The fourth heart sound results from reduced ventricular compliance producing abnormal filling.

e. False — The sound of a mitral valve prolapse is heard in mid-systole, not diastole.

86.
a. True — Although splitting of the second heart sound on inspiration is a normal finding.

b. True — The murmur of mitral regurgitation is pansystolic.

c. True — Ejection systolic murmurs may indicate pulmonary or aortic stenosis.

d. True — Mitral stenosis or tricuspid stenosis give rise to mid-diastolic murmurs.

e. False — A continuous murmur throughout systole and diastole suggests patent ductus arteriosus.

87.
a. False — Pulmonary stenosis gives rise to a murmur that is louder on inspiration.

b. False — P_2 is loud with pulmonary hypertension, but no splitting occurs.

c. True — Constrictive pericarditis limits cardiac expansion, limiting stroke volume and cardiac output.

d. False — Sinus arrhythmia is a normal finding in the young.

e. False — Reduced thoracic pressures on inspiration increase the volume of blood in the pulmonary circulation.

88.
a. False — The skin is cool and under-perfused.
b. True — Decreased vessels result in absent distal foot pulses.
c. True — Ulceration from arterial insufficiency usually occurs on the lateral aspect of the foot, on the heel or between the toes. It may, of course, occur anywhere.
d. False — These are symptoms of myocardial infarction, not peripheral vascular disease.
e. True — This is the typical appearance of skin in peripheral vascular disease.

89.
a. True — This is important to document as the patient should receive cessation advice.
b. True — Although it can't be changed, it is an indicator of cardiovascular risk.
c. True — This may interact with a number of drugs, e.g. digoxin.
d. True — These symptoms are strongly suggestive of diabetes mellitus.
e. False — Although this should be noted, it is unlikely to be directly relevant to cardiovascular disease.

90.
a. True — This is one of the cardiac causes of clubbing.
b. False — Acyanotic lesions do not cause clubbing.
c. False — Ischaemic heart disease does not cause clubbing.
d. True — This is a cyanotic heart lesion.
e. True — This is a cyanotic heart lesion.

91.
a. True — Aortic stenosis is an ejection systolic murmur.
b. True — It also frequently radiates to the axilla.
c. False — It is aortic stenosis which radiates to the carotids.
d. True — This is because it has a systolic and diastolic component.
e. False — Mitral stenosis gets louder with exercise.

92.
a. True — This is a classic examination finding, although it is often asymptomatic.
b. False — An enlarged liver or spleen may result from heart failure but not kidney.
c. False — A pulsatile liver edge is a sign of tricuspid regurgitation.
d. False — This is suggestive of portal hypertension.
e. True — This is a result of right ventricular failure and a build up of back pressure.

93.
a. False — Plain chest x-rays will rarely show signs of a pulmonary embolism.
b. True — CT using contrast medium allows precise measurement of the size of the aneurysm.

c. True — MRI with contrast media allows accurate determination of the size of the heart and the chamber volumes.
d. True — Doppler ultrasonography allows direct observation and quantification of blood flow through peripheral vessels.
e. True — Echocardiography is a highly effective technique for monitoring heart valve function.

94.
a. True — The left atrium forms the superior and left superolateral border of the heart shadow.
b. False — In the PA radiograph the heart shadow is predominantly cast by the left ventricle.
c. True — Left ventricular hypertrophy secondary to hypertension will be visible on the PA radiograph.
d. True — This is a good general guide to the size of the heart.
e. True — Left ventricular hypertrophy from the obstruction to outflow will be visible on the PA radiograph.

95.
a. False — Creatine kinase may also be released from skeletal muscle and brain.
b. True — AST is also found in liver, lung, kidney and red blood cells.
c. False — An ECG may confirm the nature of the injury and help to localize the lesion.
d. False — Lactate dehydrogenase usually peaks after 2–3 days.
e. False — Troponin is unique to cardiac cells, and so is a more specific test for myocardial injury.

96.
a. True — Echocardiography uses ultrasound to visualize the heart and its movements.
b. False — Echocardiography is the method of choice to investigate the movements of the heart and heart valves.
c. False — Echocardiography is also used to assess cardiac size.
d. False — Blood appears black, unless Doppler shift is measured, when colour is used to depict blood flow on an echocardiogram.
e. True — Doppler ultrasonography uses the changes in the reflection of sound waves from moving objects.

97.
a. False — aVL is a unipolar lead, i.e. a solitary electrode.
b. True — This enables a complete view of the heart to be taken.
c. True — This is the basis of understanding ECG rhythm strips.

211

d. True   This represents the inferior aspect of the heart.

e. False   The P wave represents atrial depolarization.

98. a. True   As a result of uncoordinated atrial activity.

b. False   This pattern is of left bundle branch block.

c. False   This dissociation is complete heart block. In second degree heart block there may be P waves without QRS complexes, but not QRS complexes without P waves.

d. False   In ventricular fibrillation the rhythm is irregular in amplitude and rate.

e. False   The QRS complex widens in left bundle branch block.

99. a. True   These are the typical features.

b. False   Hypocalcaemia prolongs the QT interval.

c. True   These are the typical features. T wave inversion in the anterior leads also commonly occurs.

d. True   These are the typical features.

e. False   The QRS complex widens in right bundle branch block.

100. a. True   Hence 0.2 s is represented by one large square.

b. False   The RR interval is used to calculate the ventricular rate.

c. False   The normal PR interval is 120–200 ms.

d. True   This explains the equal amplitude of the R and S waves.

e. False   The QT interval is normally <440 ms.

SAQ answers

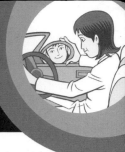

1. The functions of the heart and cardiovascular system are as follows:
   - Rapid transport of nutrients (e.g. oxygen, amino acids) and waste products (e.g. urea).
   - Hormonal control, by transporting hormones to their target organs and by secreting its own hormones, e.g. ANP.
   - Temperature regulation, by controlling heat distribution between the body core and the skin.
   - Reproduction, by producing erection of the penis.
   - Host defence, by transporting immune cells, antigens and other mediators.

2. The risk factors for ischaemic heart disease are as follows:
   - Hypercholesterolaemia – statins, dietary modification, fibrates.
   - Hypertension – β-blockers, diuretics, Ca^{2+} channel blockers, ACE inhibitors.
   - Smoking – smoking cessation products, e.g. patches, sprays, gum.
   - Diabetes mellitus – glycaemic control with oral hypoglycaemics or insulin
   - Pro-thrombotic states – aspirin.

   Other risk factors are non-modifiable, e.g. age, sex, family history, personality.

3. The four most common cardiac lesions are VSD, ASD, PDA and TGA.
   - VSD – 30% – a failure of fusion of the interventricular septum or endocardial cushions.
   - ASD – 10% – a failure of complete closure of the foramen ovale or a defect in the septum secundum.
   - PDA – 10% – a persistent opening of the ductus arteriosus allowing communication of blood between the systemic and pulmonary circulations.
   - TGA – 7% – the left ventricle pumps blood into the pulmonary trunk and the right ventricle pumps blood into the aorta (another lesion must exist to allowing mixing of the circulations, e.g. ASD).

   Bicuspid aortic valve is also a very common abnormality whereby the aortic valve has two, rather than three, cusps.

4. Varicosities on sympathetic nerves release noradrenaline (NA), which diffuses to α-adrenergic receptors on smooth muscle fibres. The G-protein coupled adrenergic receptor activates the cell via the cAMP second messenger pathway. Activation of the cell increases the intracellular calcium concentration by the following mechanisms:
   - Rapid release of Ca^{2+} from sarcoplasmic reticulum.
   - Receptor-gated Ca^{2+} channels in the sarcolemma.
   - Voltage-gated channels in the sarcolemma.
   - Caveolae, which are invaginations in the sarcolemma analogous to T tubules and are important in the smooth muscle uptake of Ca^{2+}.

5.
   a. According to Poiseuille's law: flow = (pressure difference) $\pi r^4 / \eta L$. If r doubles then r^4 increases by 16 times (2^4). This implies that flow also increases by 16 times. Thus, flow = 0.48 mL/min.
   b. η increases by 50% = η multiplied by 3/2. As η is a denominator for the flow equation then flow must change by a factor of 2/3 (i.e. flow = original flow × 2/3). Thus, flow = 0.02 mL/min.
   c. Factors contributing to the viscosity of blood are:
      - Haematocrit.
      - Plasma proteins – globulins and albumin.
      - Temperature.
      - Radius – viscosity is greater in arterioles where the marginal layer (where the cells are close to the walls) makes up a greater proportion of the lumen. Also, viscosity is less in capillaries where single file flow occurs.
      - Velocity – if flow rate is low cell agglutination occurs.
   d. Pressure difference = $P_a - P_v$ = 90 − 10 originally = 80 mmHg originally. New pressure difference = 50 − 10 = 40 mmHg now. This means that the pressure difference has halved and this implies that flow will be halved. Thus flow = 0.015 mL/min.

6.
   a. Autoregulation is the process by which the flow of blood remains constant even though the blood pressure may change. This only occurs over a limited range of pressures. The process is independent of nervous control and is due to the myogenic response and a vasodilator effect.

b. Cerebral (or renal, intestinal, coronary, skeletal muscle).

c. For small changes in pressure the perfusion of the brain will be maintained. Also autoregulation has a protective role, preventing capillary damage and oedema formation.

7. The baroreflex buffers short-term fluctuations in blood pressure. An increase in pressure causes increased stretch of the baroreceptors. This stretch increases the rate of firing of these receptors. This information is conveyed to the medulla. It results in an increase in parasympathetic drive and decreased sympathetic drive. This produces bradycardia, decreased contractility, peripheral vasodilatation, and reduced blood volumes – caused by aldosterone, angiotensin II and antidiuretic hormone (ADH) suppression. In this way the blood pressure is reduced back to normal.

A fall in blood pressure has the opposite effect.

8.

a. A vasoactive metabolite is a product of metabolism in a tissue that produces an action on the vascular smooth muscle of the supplying vessel. This action is usually relaxation of the smooth muscle producing vasodilatation.

b. Lactate, adenosine, carbon dioxide, phosphate, K^+.

c. In exercising muscle, the rise in the level of local metabolites produces vasodilatation. This increases the blood supply to the muscle and facilitates an increased metabolic rate enabling the muscle to contract.

9.

a. Stroke volume is the volume of blood ejected from the ventricle in each ventricular contraction.

b. 120 mL.

c. 50 mL.

d. 70 mL.

e. Stroke volume can be influenced by:
   • Contractility – an increase in contractility increases stroke volume.
   • Initial myocardial stretch – increased stretch (i.e. increased EDV) will increase stroke volume according to Starling's law.
   • Arterial pressure – raised arterial pressure (an increase in afterload) opposes ejection, therefore decreasing stroke volume.

f. Equations are:
   • Cardiac output (CO) = stroke volume (SV) × heart rate.
   • Stroke work (SW) = SV × arterial pressure.

10.

a. β-Blockers prevent the sympathetic stimulation of β-receptors of the heart. They have the following actions in angina:

• Decrease heart rate and therefore prolong diastole and perfusion time for the myocardium.
• Decrease oxygen demand of the myocardium by decreasing contractility and heart rate.

b. Vasospastic angina is caused by spasm of the coronary arteries and this is probably an α-adrenoreceptor-mediated action. β-Blockers have no dilatory effect on coronary arteries and so have no effect in vasospastic angina.

11.

a. Inotropic is the term used for anything that changes the contractility and therefore the force of contraction of the heart (e.g. dobutamine is a positive inotropic agent as it increases contraction). Chronotropic is the term used for any substance that alters the rate of contraction of the heart. Any agent that increases the heart rate is called a positive chronotropic agent and anything that slows the heart rate is a negative chronotropic agent.

b. An example of a positive chronotropic agent is noradrenaline.

12.

a. Muscle blood flow is increased by:
   • Metabolic vasodilatation due to vasoactive metabolites (e.g. adenosine, K^+, H^+).
   • Capillary recruitment.
   • Skeletal muscle pump, which increases venous return and, therefore, increases the pressure gradient between arterial and venous systems, driving more blood through the capillaries.
   • There may also be a central alerting response, which has a sympathetic vasodilator action on muscle vasculature and also increases cardiac output.

b. At lower temperatures paradoxical cold vasodilatation occurs in an attempt to minimize cell damage. When the skin temperature is between 10° and 15° vasoconstriction and venoconstriction occur in the hand. There is an abundance of $α_2$-receptors in the skin vessels. When the temperature falls these receptors have an increased affinity for noradrenaline. Noradrenaline causes the vascular smooth muscle to constrict, leading to vasoconstriction and, therefore, decreased flow.

13. The baroreflex that is elicited on standing leads to vaso- and venoconstriction, which counteracts the loss of blood from the thoracic compartment and the fall in cardiac output caused by standing. On continued standing, the skeletal muscle pump and the valves in the veins play the main role in aiding venous return. Contraction of extrinsic skeletal muscle compresses the vein, and this increases venous pressure. As there are valves in the veins

preventing retrograde flow then blood can only move towards the heart. This method facilitates venous return to the thoracic compartment.

The respiratory pump may also play a small role in aiding venous return. The intrathoracic pressure falls during inspiration, and this has a suction effect on the venous blood, driving it into the great veins.

14. Transmural:
- Within hours – ST elevation, T wave peaking and lengthening.
- Within 24 hours – T wave inversion, ST elevation resolves.
- Within hours or days – abnormal Q waves develop and persist, T wave inversion may persist, ST segment returns to normal.

Subendocardial:
- T wave inversion occurs.
- No Q waves form.

There may be a tachycardia, bradycardia or an abnormality of rhythm.

15. The symptoms and signs of heart failure are as follows:
- The symptoms of heart failure include: muscle fatigue, reduced exercise tolerance, dyspnoea, orthopnoea, paroxysmal nocturnal dyspnoea, haemoptysis.
- The signs of heart failure include: tachycardia, tachypnoea, elevated JVP, hepatomegaly, oedema, proteinuria, S3 heart sound.

Several compensatory mechanisms occur as a result of heart failure, the most prominent being catecholamine release, peripheral vasoconstriction and renal retention of Na^+ and water.

16. The functions of the lymphatic system are:
- Transportation of fluid and proteins. This maintains fluid balance by returning capillary filtrate to the blood.
- Absorption and transport of fat from the gastrointestinal tract.
- Presentation of foreign materials to the immune system.
- Circulation of lymphocytes.

17. Renin is an enzyme produced by the juxtaglomerular cells of the kidney. It converts angiotensinogen (from the liver) to angiotensin I. Renin production is increased by:
- A fall in afferent arterial pressure.
- Increased sympathetic activity.
- Decreased Na^+ in the macula densa.

Angiotensin converting enzyme (ACE) converts angiotensin I to angiotensin II. Angiotensin II:
- Promotes aldosterone secretion.
- Causes vasoconstriction.
- Increases cardiac contractility.

Aldosterone increases salt and water retention in the distal convoluted tubule.

18. The predominant factors causing fluid shift out of the capillary endothelium are:
- Hydrostatic pressure
  - high in the capillary at the arterial end.
  - decreased in shock.
  - increased in cardiac failure.
  - low in interstitial fluid.

The predominant factors causing fluid shift into the capillary endothelium are:
- Osmotic pressure
  - high in the capillary at the venous end.
  - decreased in renal disease, liver disease and starvation.
  - low in interstitial fluid.

Capillaries also become more permeable to protein when physically damaged.

19. Blood flow in the umbilical vessels drastically declines at birth because of:
- compression of the cord.
- vasoconstriction in response to cold, compression and catecholamines.

Pulmonary vascular resistance falls because of:
- the mechanical effect of ventilation opening the constricted alveolar vessels.
- a rising PO_2 and lowering PCO_2 causing vasodilatation.

There is an increased pulmonary blood flow, pressure drop in the right atrium and pressure rise in the left atrium. This closes the foramen ovale. The ductus venosus and ductus arteriosus close at a later stage.

20. a. In coronary artery bypass grafting:
- For LAD disease, the left internal mammary artery is detached and anastomosed distally.
- A vein is taken (usually the long saphenous), or occasionally an artery (usually the radial artery), and used to bypass other obstructions directly from the aorta.
- Improvement in symptoms is achieved in 90% of patients.
- Complications include mortality (1%) and slow occlusion of the graft.

b. In percutaneous transluminal coronary angioplasty:
- PTCA is usually used for isolated, proximal, non-calcified atheromatous plaques.
- A catheter is inserted through the femoral artery and a balloon inflated in the stenosed coronary artery to cause dilatation.
- A stent may be introduced to reduce the risk of re-stenosis.
- Complications include acute coronary occlusion and re-stenosis (occurs in 30% within 6 months).

215

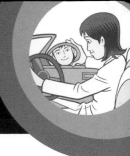

1. **Match the following descriptions of chest pain to the correct diagnosis:**

   A 5 Sharp pleuritic chest pain is typical of a pneumothorax. Spontaneous pneumothorax occurs more commonly in tall males.

   B 1 The crushing central nature of this pain is typical of a myocardial infarction, and the pattern of radiation is classic.

   C 7 Chest pain that is positional and worse on leaning forward is typical of pericarditis. This condition is a complication of SLE.

   D 8 Chest pain radiating to the back and 'tearing' in nature is classic of a thoracic dissection. There would be an asymmetry in the radial pulses associated with this condition.

   E 6 The previous episodes of chest pain were typical of angina. Since the patient now experiences pain at rest, the angina is unstable.

2. **Identify the most likely cause of shock from the scenarios below:**

   A 8 This lady has multiple risk factors, including obesity, surgery and immobility.

   B 2 This is a common presentation, an acute confusional state. The pyrexia and urinary history suggest a urinary sepsis.

   C 7 The history is typical of acute ischaemic heart disease and subsequent heart failure.

   D 4 It is likely that there is ongoing bleeding in this patient's abdomen which will require surgery.

   E 1 The symptoms are typical and the likely antigen is an anaesthetic agent or antibiotic.

3. **Identify the correct drug group from the descriptions of actions and side effects below:**

   A 5 Thiazide diuretics act on the distal convoluted tubule and prevent reabsorption of Na^+ and Cl^-.

   B 8 Low-dose aspirin has been proven to be effective in both primary and secondary prevention of ischaemic heart disease.

   C 1 β-Blockers cause a loss of peripheral β-mediated vasodilatation, causing an unopposed a vasoconstriction.

   D 4 ACE is responsible for this conversion, and ACE inhibitors therefore prevent it.

   E 9 Antibiotics prevent onset of endocarditis when there is a bacteraemia, e.g. during surgery, and are also used as treatment for established infection.

4. **Identify the arrhythmia from the ECG descriptions below:**

   A 5 The irregular pulse and absent P waves imply atrial fibrillation.

   B 6 This is a supraventricular tachycardia, but the saw-tooth appearance and rate of 150 give the diagnosis – atrial flutter with a 2:1 block.

   C 7 The only abnormality here is an increase in the PR interval, diagnostic of first degree heart block.

   D 4 This is a broad complex (arising from the ventricle), monomorphic tachycardia – ventricular tachycardia. Torsade de pointes is polymorphic.

   E 2 The PR interval is normal, but there is complete dissociation between the P waves and QRS complexes.

5. **Match the following collection of signs and symptoms to the correct diagnosis:**

A 3   The history of orthopnoea and peripheral oedema suggest a cardiac failure, in this case as a result of ischaemic heart disease.

B 4   This history suggests intermittent claudication. Diabetics are at an increased risk of peripheral vascular disease.

C 5   This is lymphoedema, and is classically non-pitting. It is likely that the pelvic surgery damaged the lymphatic vessels, predisposing to this condition.

D 7   These are most likely to be varicose veins. Being a teacher (i.e. standing for long periods) is a risk factor. The bleeding implies the swellings are superficial.

E 9   As this is unilateral, swollen and erythematous a deep venous thrombosis must be excluded. Even young adults are at risk following long haul flights.

6. **Identify from the descriptions below the correct congenital defect:**

A 4   The foramen ovale lies between the left and right atria, hence failure of this to close is an atrial septal defect.

B 3   The aorta is narrowed, hence there is decreased distal blood flow and weak femoral pulses. The murmur develops for turbulent collateral blood flow.

C 6   Both tetralogy of Fallot and transposition of the great arteries are congenital. Eisenmenger's occurs when there is reversal of a pre-existing acyanotic shunt, usually after many years.

D 10   Although ventricular septal defect is more common, atrioventricular septal defect is pathognomonic of Down syndrome.

E 9   Tetralogy of Fallot consists of pulmonary stenosis, a ventricular septal defect, right ventricular hypertrophy and an overriding aorta.

7. **Match the following signs to the correct diagnosis:**

A 8   Osler's nodes are painful transient swellings on the pulps of the fingers and toes which are indicative of endocarditis or vasculitis.

B 4   Malar flush is a peripheral cyanosis of the cheeks which indicates underlying mitral valve disease, usually mitral stenosis.

C 5   A high arched palate is one of the characteristics of Marfan syndrome, along with arachnodactyly and an increased arm span.

D 7   A collapsing pulse has a rapid rise and rapid fall. It may also be found in PDA and arteriovenous communications.

E 6   Corneal arcus are lipid deposits in the cornea. Along with xanthelasma and tendon xanthomas, these are signs of hyperlipidaemia.

8. **Match the following description of skin lesions to the correct diagnosis:**

A 1   This description is classic of a venous ulcer. The site is also highly suggestive.

B 3   As the arterial supply to this limb is compromised, this is most likely to be an arterial ulcer. Again, the site alone is highly suggestive.

C 2   The raised pearly edge is characteristic of a basal cell carcinoma.

D 9   This is most likely to be a diabetic ulcer. The foot pulses frequently remain intact as the disease predominantly affects the microvasculature. There does not appear to any neurological component.

E 8   This description is of a simple traumatic ulcer, brought on by recurrent trauma to the skin of the heel from an ill-fitting plaster cast.

9. Select the most appropriate definitive investigation for the conditions listed below:

A 7   Ventilation perfusion scans give only a probability of embolism. D dimers are non-specific. The definitive investigation is a CTPA.

B 9   The ECG will indicate whether there are any ST segment or T wave changes. Troponin I is useful but only definitive 12 hours after the onset of chest pain.

C 2   Venography identifies abnormalities in the veins. D dimers are non-specific. Venous duplex would be a good alternative.

D 3   The echocardiogram can be used to give a quantifiable measure of ventricular function and chamber size. This enables the diagnosis of heart failure to be made.

E 5   Arterial duplex gives information about the anatomy of the vessels as well as the function and distal run-off of blood.

10. Match the following descriptions to the correct cardiac murmur:

A 8   Systolic murmurs over atrioventricular valves implies incompetence. The apex is the auscultatory site of the mitral valve.

B 6   This 'machinery' sounding murmur is continuous, and found in neonates. It implies patent ductus arteriosus.

C 5   Systolic murmurs which radiate to the carotids are usually aortic stenosis. Do not confuse these with carotid bruits.

D 1   The low pitched rumbling nature of this murmur suggests a diastolic murmur. Mitral stenosis is heard best with the bell of the stethoscope.

E 7   Diastolic murmurs heard over outflow valves imply incompetence. Regurgitation of the aortic valve is very difficult to hear, so pay attention to peripheral signs, e.g. widened pulse pressure.

Index

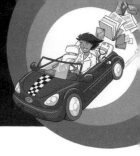

Note: Page numbers *italics* refer to diagrams and tables.